Breast and Nipple Pain II

Edited by
Kathleen Kendall-Tackett, PhD, IBCLC, FAPA

All royalties go to the
U.S. Lactation Consultant Association.

Praeclarus Press, LLC
©2019. United States Lactation Consultant Association

Praeclarus Press, LLC
2504 Sweetgum Lane
Amarillo, Texas 79124 USA
806-367-9950
www.PraeclarusPress.com

DISCLAIMER

The information contained in this publication is advisory only and is not intended to replace sound clinical judgment or individualized patient care. The author disclaims all warranties, whether expressed or implied, including any warranty as the quality, accuracy, safety, or suitability of this information for any particular purpose.

ISBN: 978-1-946665-42-3

Cover Design: Ken Tackett
Acquisition & Development: Kathleen Kendall-Tackett
Copy Editing: Kathleen Kendall-Tackett
Layout & Design: Nelly Murariu

Contents

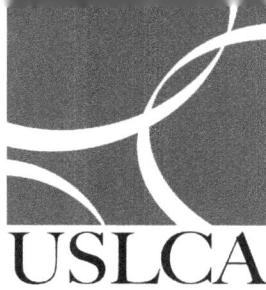

Topical Treatments Used by Breastfeeding Women to Treat Sore and Damaged Nipples

Miranda L. Buck, RN, BA, MPhil, IBCLC

Lisa H. Amir, MBBS, MMed, PhD, IBCLC, FABM, FILCA

Susan M. Donath, BSc, MEc, MA

Keywords: breastfeeding, nipple pain, nipple cream, lanolin

Background: *Nipple pain and trauma are frequent complaints of new mothers, and a variety of treatments have been proposed and investigated for efficacy. Numerous studies have examined the efficacy of nipple creams, but there is no published data describing patterns of use in breastfeeding women.*

Aim: *To describe the use of topical nipple treatments by a cohort of first-time mothers in Australia.*

Methods: *A cohort of 360 nulliparous women were recruited in Melbourne, Australia, and the question, "In* *the last week, have you used any creams or ointments on your nipples?" was included in a questionnaire on breast-feeding practices administered at 6 time points.*

Results: *In the first week after giving birth, 91% (307/336) of women used a topical treatment on their nipples. The most popular treatment was purified lanolin, with nearly three quarters of women (250/336) reporting its use. At 8 weeks postpartum, 37% (129/345) continued to use topical treatments, and 94% (320/340) of women continued to breastfeed.*

Conclusion: *Widespread use of topical nipple creams is concerning not only because it may indicate a high rate of nipple pain but also because this is a disruption to the natural environment where the newborn is establishing breastfeeding.*

Nipple pain and damage are common problems for postpartum women. Our recent study in Melbourne, Australia, found 80% of new mothers experience nipple pain in the postpartum period, with rates little changed since the first studies were conducted in the U.S. in the 1950s, despite many changes in the culture and practices of postnatal care (Buck, Amir, Cullinane, & Donath, 2014; Newton, 1952). We found no difference in pain between women who had vaginal or caesarean birth (Buck et al., 2014). Nipple pain is the second most common reason women give for weaning, and the most common for discontinuing breastfeeding before leaving hospital (Lewallen et al., 2006; Li, Fein, Chen, & Grummer-Strawn, 2008; Scott, Landers, Hughes, & Binns, 2001; Tucker, Wilson, & Samandari, 2011). Qualitative studies of women's breastfeeding experiences have consistently found that nipple pain has been an unexpectedly unpleasant burden on new mothers and which has in some cases negatively affect a woman's relationship with her baby (Amir, 2004; Kelleher, 2006; Williamson, Leeming, Lyttle, & Johnson, 2012).

The application of various preparations to soothe and heal nipples is widely recommended (Nancey, 2008; Porter & Schach, 2004; Rennie, Cowie, Hindin, & Jewell, 2009; Walker, 2013). Traditional remedies, such as onions, peppermint water, and olive oil, are also used by breastfeeding women (Akcan & Ozkiraz, 2012; Gungor et al., 2012; Sayyah Melli et al., 2007), and a recent survey of lactation instructors in the U.S. found that 65% recommend folk remedies (Schaffir & Czapla, 2012).

There are several commercially prepared nipple creams available in Australia marketed for the treatment and prevention of sore nipples. Some topical nipple treatments have been shown to reduce pain and improve healing, which may help women's experience of breastfeeding and support them in persisting to find solutions to their breastfeeding problems (Lochner, Livingston, & Judkins, 2009). However, two systematic reviews of interventions for nipple pain and trauma in breastfeeding women, Morland-Schultz and Hill (2005) and Vieira, Bachion, Mota, and Munari (2013), concluded that there is a lack of evidence as to the efficacy of any treatment because the studies that have been undertaken to date have lacked rigor.

This article presents prospective data from breastfeeding women documenting their use of nipple treatments over the first 8 postpartum weeks, using data collected in the Candida and Staphylococcus Transmission: Longitudinal Evaluation (CASTLE) study. The main aim of the CASTLE study was to determine whether Staphylococcus aureus or Candida albicans is the primary organism involved in breast thrush in lactating women, and further details are available in the published protocol and results (Amir et al., 2011, 2013).

Methods

Setting

Women were recruited from two hospitals in Melbourne, Australia: The Royal Women's Hospital (RWH), a public tertiary women's hospital in Melbourne, and Frances Perry House (FPH), a private hospital located on the same site. RWH has been accredited as Baby Friendly since 1995, and both hospitals have dedicated lactation support services. There is an onsite public pharmacy, separate from the hospital pharmacy, which sells a variety of commercial nipple ointments.

Study Sample

A prospective cohort of 360 nulliparous women was recruited between November 2009 and June 2011 (Amir et al., 2011). Eligibility criteria for the study were 18–50 years of age, nulliparity, $36 weeks pregnant at recruitment, singleton pregnancy, breastfeeding intention for at least 8 weeks postpartum, sufficient proficiency in English to complete written questionnaires and a telephone interview, and residing #16 km from Melbourne Central Business District. Criteria for exclusion were medical conditions that do not allow breastfeeding, breast reduction surgery, dermatitis on nipple during pregnancy, under care of the Women's Alcohol and Drug Service, and under care of mental health service or social worker.

Data Collection

The participants completed a questionnaire about their breastfeeding practices in hospital and at Weeks, 1, 2, 3, 4, and 8. The question asked was, "In the last week, have you used any creams or ointments on your nipples?" There were several options of types of topical treatment and a space to write any other treatments used. Any comments the participants made about why they were using the treatments during the visits were noted by the researchers; participant study numbers are presented alongside the quotes.

Results

Of the 360 women recruited at 36 weeks gestation, 14 were lost from the study, and there was data available for 346; 154 from RWH and 192 from FPH. The mean age was 32.7 years with a range of 19–44, and the caesarean rate was 45% (156/346). This was a highly educated sample of women, with 77% (267/346) having a tertiary degree or higher.

The majority of the women were married or living with their partner (332/346). The mean intention to breastfeed was 9.7 months (range 1–24 months). At 8 weeks, 80% of the babies were fully breastfed, and 94% (320/340) were receiving any breast milk.

In the first week after birth, 91% (307/336) of women were using some form of nipple treatment (see Table 1). By far the most popular choice of treatment was purified lanolin; 74% (250/336) of postpartum women were using lanolin at Week 1, almost half were using it after 4 weeks and at 8 weeks 26% (89/345). Overall, 18 distinct commercial treatments were found to be in use, and one woman used olive oil. Early in the study period, Weeks 1–4, hydrogel dressings were used by up to 12% (40/336) of women for the treatment of cracked and damaged nipples, but use of hydrogel dressings had been discontinued by 8 weeks.

The following comments are examples of the notes taken by researchers during their visits with the participants to collect data:

> Between wk 4 & 5 postpartum participant had stabbing breast pain. Infant had white coating on tongue. Participant's sister-in-law (midwife) suggested she may have nipple thrush. Participant went to pharmacist who also suggested nipple thrush and gave participant Daktarin gel [miconazole]. Participant used Daktarin gel for 3 days on her nipple every feed. The breast pain went away after this time. White coating also disappeared from baby's tongue. (Participant FPH190)

3 wk ago participant thought she had nipple thrush. She thought her baby had oral thrush. She brought her baby to GP who did not diagnose oral thrush but prescribed Daktarin gel for mother's nipples and baby's mouth as a precaution. Participant used Daktarin on her nipples for a week and intermittently since then. (Participant RWH82)

Table 1. Treatments Used By Week

Type of Treatment	Hospital (n = 338) n (%)	Week 1 (n = 336) n (%)	Week 2 (n = 336) n (%)	Week 3 (n = 326) n (%)	Week 4 (n = 323) n (%)	Week 8 (n = 345) n (%)
Purified lanolin	103 (30)	250 (74)	220 (65)	178 (56)	155 (48)	89 (26)
Antifungal cream	0	1 (0.3)	3 (1)	1 (0.3)	2 (1)	1 (0.3)
Antifungal gel	0	1 (0.3)	8 (2)	12 (4)	17 (5)	26 (8)
Gentian Violet	0	0	0	0	0	2 (1)
Antibiotic ointment	1 (0.3)	0	0	2 (1)	0	1 (0.3)
Combination ointment	1 (0.3)	0	2 (1)	6 (2)	4 (1)	1 (0.3)
Hydrogel dressing	11 (3)	40 (12)	31 (9)	18 (6)	17 (5)	0
Lucas' Pawpaw Ointment[a]	2 (1)	6 (2)	2 (1)	6 (2)	1 (0.3)	6 (2)
Other[b]	4 (1)	9 (3)	6 (2)	11 (3)	9 (3)	3 (1)

[a]Lucas' Pawpaw Ointment is an Australian product containing petroleum jelly and *Carica papaya*.
[b]A number of other creams were used by individual women: Aveda Nipple Care Balm, Bepanthen, Betadine Antiseptic Ointment, Calendula cream, Gentian Violet (two women in week 8), Mustela Nursing Comfort Balm, Nuk Nipple Cream, olive oil, Palmer's Cocoa Butter Nursing Cream, phytoseptic (Golden Seal; *Hydrastis Canadensis*), QV cream, Vaseline, Weleda Nipple Care Cream.

Participant had stabbing breast pain in right breast this week. Given Daktarin oral gel. GP told her to use it on the right nipple only. Not putting it in the baby's mouth. (Participant FPH104)

GP prescribed antibiotics and Daktarin gel for suspected mastitis. (Participant RWH110)

Antifungal gel usage was observed as an increasing trend over the duration of the study, from one woman in Week 1 to 26 (8%) in week 8. This rising prevalence was not seen for combination, antibiotic, or non-medicated creams. In keeping with this rise in antifungal use over the study period, two women had begun to use Gentian Violet by the end of the study. Over the entire study, antifungal gels were used by 47 (14%) individual women. Two women used antifungal gel from Weeks 2 to 8, and four women (1%) from Weeks 3 to 8.

Discussion

The strengths of this study are that it was a prospective study with high retention, and the women reported all usage of topical nipple treatments in the first 8 weeks of breastfeeding. There was a sharp increase in use of treatments between data collected in hospital and at the end of Week 1. It is possible that when they were presented with the list of creams that may have been used in the first few days after birth, it suggested to the women that they should or could be using a cream and therefore artificially inflated the prevalence.

This study is not able to evaluate how successful the strategies were or why the women chose those particular products, and we did not ask if they were advised to use them by a health care professional. We did not specifically ask the women if they had been applying breast milk to their nipples or about their hygiene practices generally. Many of the participants were recruited in the breast-feeding education classes provided by the hospital, and lanolin was likely to have been recommended in those classes and also by the midwives on the antenatal wards (A. Moorhead, Clinical Midwife Consultant, personal communication, June 16, 2014).

Nipple Care During the Early Postpartum Period

Recommendations for nipple care vary enormously and can be conflicting; women are variously advised to wash their nipples with soap, or with nothing but plain water, to apply breast milk, to apply creams, of the benefits of a moist healing environment, or to air dry their nipples and frequently change breast pads to prevent dampness (Australian Breastfeeding Association, 2011; Newman & Kernerman, 2009; Walker, 2013). This is the first study to prospectively explore the use of topical therapies by breast-feeding women. Over the 8 weeks of the study, a pattern of almost universal use of some form of treatment was seen in the early weeks decreasing over time.

Intervention Strategies for Mothers With Sore Nipples

Most women experience some initial difficulties with pain and damage during the early days of breastfeeding. When pain and damage interfere with the establishment of breastfeeding, specific and holistic treatment is warranted. Brodribb (2012) recommends the following principles of general management:

- Offer the least sore nipple first.

- Induce letdown before bringing the baby to the breast.

- Suggest baby-led latch or an upright koala hold.

- Encourage small frequent feeds to prevent engorgement.

- Apply warm compresses immediately post feeds for 5 minutes.

- A moist wound healing environment between feeds will reduce pain and speed wound healing.

Wound Healing and Lanolin Use

Wound healing can be described in terms of three stages—inflammation, granulation, and remodeling—and is influenced by many factors including age, sex hormones, medications, stress, and nutrition (Guo & DiPietro, 2010; Kondo & Ishida, 2010). The lactating woman's nipple is a particularly challenging area to support in terms of healing because of the necessity to keep using the tissue and concerns for the infant's safety when topical medications may be ingested.

Nearly three quarters of this cohort applied purified lanolin to their nipples in the first week of breastfeeding. Lanolin is extracted from sheep wool and is chemically a wax "ultrarefined" to remove free lanolin alcohols to a level lower than 1.5% (Abou-Dakn, Fluhr, Gensch, & Wöckel, 2011). It has been successfully used for several therapeutic purposes including healing anal fissures in children and preventing lip breakdown in adults undergoing chemotherapy (Büyükyavuz, Savas, & Duman, 2010; Santos et al., 2013). Chvapil, Gaines, and Gilman (1988), in their detailed study of lanolin and wound healing in piglets, suggested that lanolin may promote an inflammatory response, which encourages reepithelialization. On a cellular level, the promotion of healing is better than a plain gauze dressing.

Purified lanolin provides a moist healing environment and has been compared to other treatments for sore nipples and shown to be helpful in reducing pain and supporting healing, but most studies have been small (Coca & Abrao, 2008; Gungor et al., 2012; Vieira et al., 2013). Although concerns have been voiced that lanolin may be associated with an increased risk of infection (Sasaki, Pinkerton, & Leipelt, 2014), Dennis, Schottle, Hodnett, and McQueen (2012) found that in their Toronto study of 151 women, those using lanolin had higher breastfeeding rates at 12 weeks postpartum and had a significantly more pleasant experience of breastfeeding than those using an all-purpose combined cream.

Increased Use of Antifungals During the First 8 Weeks

Over the course of the first 8 weeks postpartum, women's use of lanolin slowly fell, but antifungal treatments were increasingly popular, with 8% (29/346) using some form of antifungal in Week 8, including two women who were prescribed Gentian Violet. Gentian Violet is recommended on the RWH protocol for the treatment of nipple thrush, as a 0.5% aqueous paint, to be applied after breast-feeding twice a day for up to 7 days, when miconazole, nystatin, and fluconazole treatments have failed (RWH, 2013). Comments made by the women on why they were using antifungal gel suggests that some of the use may be preventive and used in tandem with antibiotics for mastitis. Four women (1%) reported using antifungal gel for 4 weeks and two women for six weeks. This prolonged use of antifungal gel is concerning.

Other Topical Treatments

Lucas' Pawpaw ointment is an Australian product containing petroleum jelly and Carica Papaya extract and was used by small numbers of women at each time point. Several of the creams used, Palmer's, QV, and Bepanthen, are petroleum-based, and some contain polyethylene glycol ethers, which are not recommended for use on broken skin and known to be irritants (Andersen, 1999). Phytoseptic ointment, Weleda, and calendula creams were also used by women in this study. There has been an increasing interest in the use of plant-based extracts in wound healing, and several studies have been published that are promising and suggest that many traditional herbal remedies may be useful.

Süntar et al. (2011), for example, found that a preparation of sage and oregano oils "displays remarkable wound healing activity" and is both bactericidal and fungicidal. Cinnamon, lemongrass, and peppermint have also suggested as potential novel therapies (Liakos et al., 2014; Sayyah Melli et al., 2007). Coconut oil has been shown to be antifungal, antibacterial, used safely in topical massage of premature babies, and as a useful treatment in the wound healing of burns (Das, Rahman, Chowdhury, Hoq, & Deb, 2013; Nangia, Paul, Chawla, & Deorari, 2008; Ogbolu, Oni, Daini, & Oloko, 2007; Srivastava & Durgaprasad, 2008; Valizadeh, Hosseini, Jafarabadi, & Ajoodanian, 2012).

Hydrogel Dressings

Hydrogel dressings were used by 12% of the women, but use had been discontinued by Week 8 of the study. These dressings are expensive; there has been some concerns raised that although they may reduce pain, they may increase the risk of infection (Benbow & Vardy-White, 2004; Brent, Rudy, Redd, Rudy, & Roth, 1998), and they are not recommended by Vieira et al. (2013) in their systematic review.

Concerns About the Use of Topical Treatments

The mother's breast is the native environment of the newborn baby, and skin-to-skin contact between neonate and mother at birth initiates a cascade of primitive behaviors and reflexes that supports the establishment of both breastfeeding and the mother–infant bond (Barry & Tighe, 2013; Bigelow, Littlejohn, Bergman, & McDonald, 2010; Bramson et al., 2010; Colson, Meek, & Hawdon, 2008; Mahmood, Jamal, & Khan, 2011; Widström et al., 2011). How well the newborn baby initially seeks out and attaches to the nipple may influence the course of breastfeeding, and this in turn is influenced by the sensory environment at the breast. The smell and feel of their mother's skin varies by birthing and hygiene practices and also according to secretions of Montgomery glands on the nipple (Doucet, Soussignan, Sagot, & Schaal, 2009, 2012; Preer, Pisegna, Cook, Henri, & Philipp, 2013). It is of some concern that such widespread use of topical creams was found not only because it may indicate a high frequency of nipple pain but also because this is a disruption to the natural environment and experience of breastfeeding for the baby, the consequences of which are unknown.

Conclusion

Nipple pain is a key risk to the continuation breastfeeding and also causes considerable distress to new mothers. The use of topical treatments, notably purified lanolin, for the prevention and treatment of nipple problems in breastfeeding is very common, but what this means for the experience of infants at the breast and the establishment of successful breastfeeding is unknown. Further research is required to establish both an effective intervention for the prevention of nipple trauma and timely treatment of damaged and sore nipples, which need careful evaluation.

References

Abou-Dakn, M., Fluhr, J. W., Gensch, M., & Wöckel, A. (2011). Positive effect of HPA lanolin versus expressed breastmilk on painful and damaged nipples during lactation. *Skin Pharmacology and Physiology, 24*(1), 27–35.

Akcan, A. B., & Ozkiraz, S. (2012). An unusual traditional practice for damaged nipples during lactation. *Breastfeeding Medicine, 7,* 319.

Amir, L. H. (2004). Test your knowledge. Nipple pain in breastfeeding. *Australian Family Physician, 33*(1–2), 44–45.

Amir, L. H., Cullinane, M., Garland, S. M., Tabrizi, S. N., Donath, S. M., Bennett, C. M., . . . Payne, M. S. (2011). The role of micro–organisms (Staphylococcus aureus and Candida albicans) in the pathogenesis of breast pain and infection in lactating women: Study protocol. *BMC Pregnancy and Childbirth, 11,* 54.

Amir, L. H., Donath, S. M., Garland, S. M., Tabrizi, S. N., Bennett, C. M., Cullinane, M., & Payne, M. S. (2013). Does Candida and/or Staphylococcus play a role in nipple and breast pain in lactation? A cohort study in Melbourne, Australia. *BMJ Open, 3*(3), e002351.

Andersen, F. A. (1999). Final report on the safety assessment of Ceteth 21, 22, 23, 24, 25, 26, 210, 212, 214, 215, 216, 220, 224, 225, 230, and, 245. *International Journal of Toxicology, 18*(2 Suppl.), 1–8.

Australian Breastfeeding Association. (2011). *Sore/cracked nipples.* Retrieved from https://www.breastfeeding.asn.au/bf-info/common-concerns%E2%80%93mum/sore-cracked-nipples

Barry, M., & Tighe, S. M. (2013). Facilitating effective initiation of breastfeeding—A review of the recent evidence base. *British Journal of Midwifery, 21*(5), 312–315.

Benbow, M., & Vardy-White, C. (2004). Study into the effectiveness of MOTHERMATES. *British Journal of Midwifery, 12*(4), 244–248.

Bigelow, A. E., Littlejohn, M., Bergman, N., & McDonald, C. (2010). The relation between early mother–infant skin-to-skin contact and later maternal sensitivity in South African mothers of low birth weight infants. *Infant Mental Health Journal, 31*(3), 358–377.

Bramson, L., Lee, J. W., Moore, E., Montgomery, S., Neish, C., Bahjri, K., & Melcher, C. L. (2010). Effect of early skin-to-skin mother–infant contact during the first 3 hours following birth on exclusive breastfeeding during the maternity hospital stay. *Journal of Human Lactation, 26*(2), 130–137.

Brent, N., Rudy, S. J., Redd, B., Rudy, T. E., & Roth, L. A. (1998). Sore nipples in breastfeeding women: A clinical trial of wound dressings vs conventional care. *Archives of Pediatric and Adolescent Medicine, 152*(11), 1077–1082.

Brodribb, W. (2012). *Breastfeeding management in Australia: Victoria, Australia*: Australian Breastfeeding Association.

Buck, M. L., Amir, L. H., Cullinane, M., & Donath, S. M. (2014). Nipple pain, damage and vasospasm in the first 8 weeks postpartum. *Breastfeeding Medicine, 9*(2), 56–62.

Büyükyavuz, B. I., Savas, Ç., & Duman, L. (2010). Efficacy of lanolin and bovine type I collagen in the treatment of childhood anal fissures: A prospective, randomized, controlled clinical trial. *Surgery Today, 40*(8), 752–756.

Chvapil, M., Gaines, J. A., & Gilman, T. (1988). Lanolin and epidermal growth factor in healing of partial-thickness pig wounds. *Journal of Burn Care & Research, 9*(3), 279–284.

Coca, K. P., & Abrao, A. C. F. V. (2008). An evaluation of the effect of lanolin in healing nipple injuries. *Acta Paulista de Enfermagem, 21*(1), 11–16.

Colson, S. D., Meek, J. H., & Hawdon, J. M. (2008). Optimal positions for the release of primitive neonatal reflexes stimulating breastfeeding. *Early Human Development, 84*(7), 441–449.

Das, S. R., Rahman, A. M., Chowdhury, A. A., Hoq, M. M., & Deb, S. R. (2013). Effect of application of sunflower and coconut oils over the skin of low birth weight babies in prevention of nosocomial infection. *Journal of Dhaka Medical College, 21*(2), 160–165.

Dennis, C.-L., Schottle, N., Hodnett, E., & McQueen, K. (2012). An all-purpose nipple ointment versus lanolin in treating painful damaged nipples in breastfeeding women: A randomized controlled trial. *Breastfeeding Medicine, 7*(6), 473–479.

Doucet, S., Soussignan, R., Sagot, P., & Schaal, B. (2009). The secretion of areolar (Montgomery's) glands from lactating women elicits selective, unconditional responses in neonates. *PLoS One, 4*(10), e7579.

Doucet, S., Soussignan, R., Sagot, P., & Schaal, B. (2012). An overlooked aspect of the human breast: Areolar glands in relation with breastfeeding pattern, neonatal weight gain, and the dynamics of lactation. *Early Human Development, 88*(2), 119–128.

Gungor, A., Oguz, S., Vurur, G., Gencer, M., Uysal, A., Hacivelioglu, S., . . . Cosar, E. (2012). Comparison of olive oil and lanolin in the prevention of sore nipples in nursing mothers [Letter to the editor]. *Breastfeeding Medicine, 8*(3), 334–335.

Guo, S., & DiPietro, L. A. (2010). Factors affecting wound healing. *Journal of Dental Research, 89*(3), 219–229.

Kelleher, C. M. (2006). The physical challenges of early breastfeeding. *Social Science & Medicine, 63*(10), 2727–2738.

Kondo, T., & Ishida, Y. (2010). Molecular pathology of wound healing. *Forensic Science International, 203*(1–3), 93–98.

Lewallen, L. P., Dick, M. J., Flowers, J., Powell, W., Zickefoose, K. T., Wall, Y. G., & Price, Z. M. (2006). Breastfeeding support and early cessation. *Journal of Obstetric, Gynecologic, ands Neonatal Nursing, 35*(2), 166–172.

Li, R., Fein, S. B., Chen, J., & Grummer-Strawn, L. M. (2008). Why mothers stop breastfeeding: Mothers' self-reported reasons for stopping during the first year. *Pediatrics, 122*(Supp. 2), S69–S76.

Liakos, I., Rizzello, L., Scurr, D. J., Pompa, P. P., Bayer, I. S., & Athanassiou, A. (2014). All-natural composite wound dressing films of essential oils encapsulated in sodium alginate with antimicrobial properties. *International Journal of Pharmaceutics, 463*(2), 137–145.

Lochner, J. E., Livingston, C. J., & Judkins, D. Z. (2009). Clinical inquiries: Which interventions are best for alleviating nipple pain in nursing mothers? *Journal of Family Practice, 58*(11), 612a–612c.

Mahmood, I., Jamal, M., & Khan, N. (2011). Effect of mother-infant early skin-to-skin contact on breastfeeding status: A randomized controlled trial. *Journal of the College of Physicians and Surgeons Pakistan, 21*(10), 601–605.

Morland-Schultz, K., & Hill, P. D. (2005). Prevention of and therapies for nipple pain: A systematic review. *Journal of Obstetric, Gynecologic & Neonatal Nursing, 34*(4), 428–437.

Nancey, J. S. (2008). Breastfeeding 'struggles': Care and management for sore and cracked nipples. *MIDIRS Midwifery Digest, 18*(4), 561–564.

Nangia, S., Paul, V., Chawla, D., & Deorari, A. (2008). Topical coconut oil application reduces transepidermal water loss in preterm very low birth weight neonates: A randomized clinical trial. *Pediatrics, 121*(Suppl. 2), S139.

Newman, J., & Kernerman, E. (2009). *Sore nipples.* Retrieved from http://www.nbci.ca/index.php?option=com_content&id=48:sore-nipples&Itemid=17

Newton, N. (1952). Nipple pain and nipple damage: Problems in the management of breast feeding. *Journal of Pediatrics, 41*(4), 411–423.

Ogbolu, D., Oni, A., Daini, O., & Oloko, A. (2007). In vitro antimicrobial properties of coconut oil on Candida species in Ibadan, Nigeria. *Journal of Medicinal Food, 10*(2), 384–387.

Porter, J., & Schach, B. (2004). Treating sore, possibly infected nipples. *Journal of Human Lactation, 20*(2), 221–222.

Preer, G., Pisegna, J. M., Cook, J. T., Henri, A.-M., & Philipp, B. L. (2013). Delaying the bath and in-hospital breastfeeding rates. *Breastfeeding Medicine, 8*, 485–490.

Rennie, A. M., Cowie, J., Hindin, P. K., & Jewell, S. (2009). The management of nipple pain and/or trauma associated with breastfeeding. *Best Practice, 13*(4), 17–20.

Santos, P. S., Tinoco-Araujo, J. E., Souza, L. M., Ferreira, R., Ikoma, M. R., Razera, A. P., & Santos, M. M. (2013). Efficacy of HPA Lanolin® in treatment of lip alterations related to chemotherapy. *Journal of Applied Oral Science, 21*(2), 163–166.

Sasaki, B. C., Pinkerton, K., & Leipelt, A. (2014). Does lanolin use increase the risk for infection in breastfeeding women? *Clinical Lactation, 5*(1), 28–32.

Sayyah Melli, M., Rashidi, M. R., Delazar, A., Madarek, E., Kargar Maher, M. H., Ghasemzadeh, A., . . . Tahmasebi, Z. (2007). Effect of peppermint water on prevention of nipple cracks in lactating primiparous women: A randomized controlled trial. *International Breastfeeding Journal, 2*, 7.

Schaffir, J., & Czapla, C. (2012). Survey of lactation instructors on folk traditions in breastfeeding. *Breastfeeding Medicine, 7*(4), 230–233.

Scott, J. A., Landers, M. C. G., Hughes, R. M., & Binns, C. W. (2001). Psychosocial factors associated with the abandonment of breastfeeding prior to hospital discharge. *Journal of Human Lactation, 17*(1), 24–30.

Srivastava, P., & Durgaprasad, S. (2008). Burn wound healing property of Cocos nucifera: An appraisal. Indian *Journal of Pharmacology, 40*(4), 144–146.

Süntar, I., Akkol, E. K., Keles, H., Oktem, A., Baser, K. H. C., & Yesilada, E. (2011). A novel wound healing ointment: A formulation of Hypericum perforatum oil and sage and oregano essential oils based on traditional Turkish knowledge. *Journal of Ethnopharmacology, 134*(1), 89–96.

The Royal Women's Hospital. (2013). *Breast & nipple thrush. Retrieved* from http://www.thewomens.org.au/uploads/downloads/HealthProfessionals/PGP_PDFs/ March_2013/Breast_and_Nipple_Thrush.pdf

Tucker, C. M., Wilson, E. K., & Samandari, G. (2011). Infant feeding experiences among teen mothers in North Carolina: Findings from a mixed-methods study. *International Breastfeeding Journal, 6,* 14.

Valizadeh, S., Hosseini, M. B., Jafarabadi, M. A., & Ajoodanian, N. (2012). The effects of massage with coconut and sunflower oils on oxygen saturation of premature infants with respiratory distress syndrome treated with nasal continuous positive airway pressure. *Journal of Caring Sciences, 1*(4), 191–199.

Vieira, F., Bachion, M. M., Mota, D. D., & Munari, D. B. (2013). A systematic review of the interventions for nipple trauma in breastfeeding mothers. *Journal of Nursing Scholarship, 45*(2), 116–125.

Walker, M. (2013). Are there any cures for sore nipples? *Clinical Lactation, 4*(3), 106–115.

Widström, A. M., Lilja, G., Aaltomaa-Michalias, P., Dahllöf, A., Lintula, M., & Nissen, E. (2011). Newborn behaviour to locate the breast when skin-to-skin: A possible method for enabling early self-regulation. *Acta Paediatrica, 100*(1), 79–85.

Williamson, I., Leeming, D., Lyttle, S., & Johnson, S. (2012). 'It should be the most natural thing in the world': Exploring firsttime mothers' breastfeeding difficulties in the UK using audiodiaries and interviews. *Maternal & Child Nutrition, 8*(4), 434–447.

Ethics: This study was approved by the La Trobe University Human Ethics Committee (06–078), Human Research Ethics Committee of The Royal Women's Hospital (06/41); Human Research Ethics Committee of the University of Melbourne (1033949), and Medical Advisory Committee at Frances Perry House.

Funding: This study received financial support from the National Health and Medical Research Council (project grant 541907, equipment grant, Health Professional Training Fellowship [LHA]), Helen Macpherson Smith Trust, Faculty Research Grant, Faculty of Health Sciences, La Trobe University. MLB has a Faculty of Health Sciences, La Trobe University, Dean's Scholarship.

Help for Sore Nipples

Below are examples of some of the advice mothers get about treating sore nipples. Some advice in these videos is helpful. Much of this advice is contradictory or outdated. And one video even recommends formula feeds for overcoming sore nipples!

https://www.youtube.com/watch?v=6BC5zfdZgPE

https://www.youtube.com/watch?v=bkk_YW2SY2k

https://www.youtube.com/watch?v=beQAaHqT_6Q

https://www.youtube.com/watch?v=WBgcon8pMeE

https://www.youtube.com/watch?v=ksH9H4AStmM

https://www.youtube.com/watch?v=vsluv5s8VXE

Family and Medical Leave Act Guide From the National Partnership for Women and Family

The National Partnership for Women & Families has released the seventh edition of the Guide to the Family and Medical Leave Act, available in both English and Spanish. The guide is a comprehensive explanation of the FMLA that aims to make the law more accessible and help individuals navigate its protections and the adjustments made to it over the years.

Source: USBC

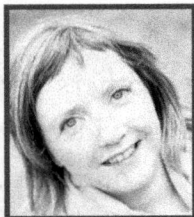

Miranda L. Buck, RN, BA, MPhil, IBCLC, is a neonatal nurse and International Board Certified Lactation Consultant. She works as a lactation consultant at The Royal Women's Hospital in Melbourne and is a PhD candidate at the Judith Lumley Centre, La Trobe University. A recipient of the dean's scholarship in 2010, Ms. Buck is investigating women's experiences of breastfeeding problems and nipple pain using data collected in the CASTLE project.

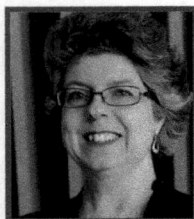

Lisa H. Amir, MBBS, MMed, PhD, IBCLC, FABM, FILCA, is a general practitioner and lactation consultant.

She works in breastfeeding medicine at The Royal Women's Hospital and in private practice. She is a principal research fellow at the Judith Lumley Centre, La Trobe University, Australia. She is the author of over 60 peer-reviewed articles and the editor-in-chief of International Breastfeeding Journal.

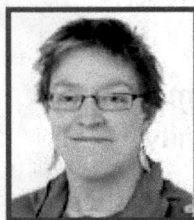

Susan M. Donath, BSc, MEc, MA, is a senior biostatistician and epidemiologist with extensive experience in the design and analysis of quantitative health-related research, perinatal epidemiology, and clinical trials. Susan is an author of more than 130 publications in refereed journals, 70 of which have been published in the last 5 years. These publications cover a wide spectrum of research areas, including laboratory-based, clinical, public health, nursing, and allied health research projects, predominantly in pediatric and women's health.

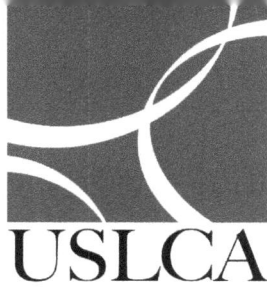

USLCA

Revisiting Nipple and Breast Pain

A Conversation With Anne Eglash, MD

Barbara Robertson

Keywords: breastfeeding, lactation, nipple pain, breast pain, vasospasm, biofilm, mastitis, yeast, probiotics, IBCLC, breast dysbiosis

Barbara D. Robertson and Dr. Anne Eglash discuss Dr. Eglash's latest thoughts on breast and nipple pain. Unresolved breast and nipple pain are one of the top reasons for early weaning. Dr. Eglash has a breastfeeding medical practice and helps mothers frequently to help resolve their chronic breast and nipple pain. Old treatments are discussed in the context of new research findings and new treatment possibilities are explored.

Barbara Robertson recently had an opportunity to speak with Anne Eglash, MD, IBCLC, FABM, about breast and nipple pain. Anne obtained her International Board Certified Lactation Consultant (IBCLC) certification in 1994, the same year she cofounded the Academy of Breastfeeding Medicine with 11 other physicians. The main purpose for starting this organization was to educate physicians and other health professionals about breastfeeding.

This was based on my experience with my first two kids before 1994 of not finding any help in the medical field. I found help from other people but not physicians and nurses. I feel like my life has been dedicated to physician and other health professional education in breastfeeding.

Dr. Eglash is a clinical professor with the University of Wisconsin School of Medicine and Public Health, in the Department of Family Medicine. She is a family physician and has been a board-certified lactation consultant since 1994. She is the medical director of the outpatient lactation program at Meriter Hospital and the medical director of the University of Wisconsin Lactation Clinic, which is a teaching breastfeeding clinic. She is a cofounder of the Academy of Breastfeeding Medicine and is the co-medical director and cofounder of the Mothers' Milk Bank of the Western Great Lakes. She is also the founder and president of The Milk Mob (www.themilkmob.org), a nonprofit organization dedicated to outpatient breastfeeding education for health professionals and other community breastfeeding supporters.

She has published many peer-reviewed articles on breastfeeding medicine and sits on the editorial board for Breastfeeding Medicine. She hosts and produces a free breastfeeding medicine podcast series available on iTunes.

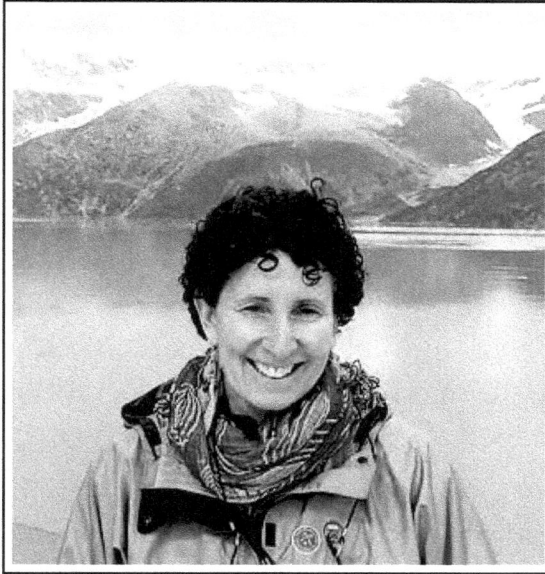

Figure 1. Anne Eglash

BR: Thank you for taking the time to do this interview. There is a lot of confusion about breast pain and nipple pain. The more we can try to help IBCLCs understand the difference in types of pain and possible treatments, I think it will be helping a lot of moms and babies. There seems to be a lot of reluctance in the medical profession in my area to use science when diagnosing breast and nipple pain. What kind of medical testing can be done to help diagnose pain?

AE: The big thing about diagnosing is really just like anything else in medicine. The first thing that people have to do is listen to the patient. Ninety percent of the information I'm going to get about that patient to make the decision is going to come directly from what the patient tells me. So, it's not just about the exam. I mean the exam is important definitely, but it's like anything else, you need to listen to the patient. The physicians don't know the questions to ask until they understand the problem. So, physicians cannot evaluate and make a diagnosis about breast pain when they don't know anything about it. What they need is education. Just like if someone comes in to me with a headache and I know nothing about headaches. What kind of questions am I going to ask? I don't know. What's important? Is it important that it is pounding? The first thing that has to happen is that doctors need education about breastfeeding.

If you're going to make a diagnosis of breast pain, you have to understand the pattern of the pain, when the mother is having pain, does it happen at the onset of latch, does the latch hurt at all, does the pain happen after the feeding, is it always associated with blanching, is it never associated with blanching, has there been mastitis, plugged ducts? There is a whole list of questions that have to be asked in order for me to determine what is causing the breast pain. Then comes the physical exam: looking at the breast, looking to see if there are sores, any evidence of infection, any redness or swelling, any abscess, is the breast tender? I do a manual expression to see if that causes pain, a breast palpation to see if that is tender. The breast is not going to be tender necessarily if it's vasospasm or latch pain. If a woman has a dysbiosis, where there is a bacterial imbalance in the ducts, her breast is generally going to be really tender. Or if she has mastitis, she will be tender.

Then the next thing I would do, if I think it is warranted, is a breast milk culture. And I do the culture a very specific way. There is a protocol that I have at the University of Washington lab. I make sure they do sensitivities on different antibiotics to see what antibiotics the bacteria are sensitive to. And then I just put all that information together. And, of course, I'm watching breastfeeding as part of the exam. I look at the babies to see if they have any lip or tongue tie, torticollis, or thrush. Then I watch the babies nurse to make sure that looks okay. I ask moms to bring their pump to make sure they are not suffering pump trauma. This kind of evaluation, which is another limitation to doctors, can take me an hour to evaluate a patient. Because you have to examine mom, examine baby, and evaluate nursing . . . (you have to) find an hour for a medical problem that is really difficult.

BR: So back to my question about what type of testing can be done to evaluate nipple pain. The testing, that's not really the problem. The problem is the doctors are unfamiliar with breastfeeding, period, to even ask the right questions. The idea that somehow bacterial or yeast testing is the missing link really is not the problem. It starts with a basic lack of breastfeeding knowledge to begin with from the get go.

AE: There is no specific test to know what is causing the pain. It all has to do with health history and physical exams. Most of the data is from the dairy industry, about the concerns about bacteria in the dairy industry.

BR: Side question . . . Does the dairy industry struggle with yeast the same way we do?

AE: No. And the reason why is because (the pain) is not yeast. This is a bacterial imbalance. They don't worry about yeast. I don't worry about yeast. Yeast is usually not the issue. This is usually bacterial imbalance.

BR: That's what I have believed for years by reading the literature and talking with other professionals. Is that yeast is overly diagnosed (**AE:** Yes.), and we are not getting to the real problem. And then with yeast moms are told they have to boil their pumps parts, their pacifiers, nursing bras, and they have to sterilize their bottles. And I think about a vaginal yeast infection, you take your medication, whatever you are going to do, and you are done. You don't boil your underwear or throw them away. You just wash them in the wash, put them back on, and the yeast doesn't come back.

AE: Right.

BR: My conclusions about yeast have been, and you can tell me right or wrong, that if I if my yeast is in balance, we all have yeast all the time, then you can't give me a yeast overgrowth.

AE: You can have a yeast overgrowth. You can have an imbalance.

BR: For sure, but if my yeast is in balance, you can't "give" me a yeast overgrowth? My mom with yeast infection can't give it to me?

AE: Yes, I think so. For example, a man who has a groin infection, like Candida, he will pass yeast to his sexual partner. A woman who has a vaginal yeast infection, the man might start to get itchy and get yeast in the crevices of his penis or scrotum. So, you can actually pass it.

BR: Can you tell me more about that? Because it seems to me you're either in balance or out of balance. And if your yeast is in balance, how can another person give you a yeast imbalance?

AE: I don't have an answer to that. I don't know.

BR: You have just seen it professionally and it happens?

AE: Exactly. Yes, and it might be that that person just eats a lot of sugar, or has diabetes, so the partners are susceptible. It's a good point you are making. We all reach a certain balance with our yeast, and when most women have a vaginal yeast infection, the majority of men do not get jock itch. So, this is a really good point you are bringing up. The researchers in Spain talk about this whole issue, that the breast milieu is a very inhospitable place for Candida to grow, so it makes sense that Candida wouldn't grow in the breast, and they also talk about how there is this relationship between Candida and Staph epi, which is the predominate bacteria in breast milk. So, whenever a woman lactates, her milk ducts are populated by a very complicated microbiome. There are lots of different bacteria, probiotics, and Staph epidermatitis. Staph epi is the bacterium that is on every one's skin, and it highly populates the breast. The theory is when that Staph epi comes in contact with the yeast that is in the baby's mouth, that Staph epi changes its behavior. It turns on certain genes and the bacteria forms a biofilm. And have you ever seen women who have chronic breast pain and they get that mucky white stuff on their nipples?

BR: Yes, it's crusty. And from what I have heard, from Marsha Walker and other people, one should wash with soap and water to help clear that film.

AE: It not a yeast infection. But everyone thinks that it is. It's not just on the nipples, it's in the ducts. So, what happens is Staph epi is forming that biofilm as an umbrella to protect itself from the body's own antibacterial factors. Some of the factors in the breast milk are there to serve the breast itself, to keep the breast healthy. So, when Staph epi is exposed to the Candida, the Staph epi can turn on certain genes that allow it to form that biofilm. And that is why I think this whole history of "Oh, you have yeast and your baby has yeast because you have yeast." Well, it's not that. It's the formation of what I would call a dysbiosis, a term that means bad microbiotic environment. The bacterial environment is off.

Suddenly you have the bacteria milieu going awry, very much like bacterial vaginosis. I've been looking at bacterial vaginosis . . . what we have found is women with a history of bacterial vaginosis also have low vitamin D. Low D levels are associated with recurrent bacterial vaginosis. I have gotten all my patients who suffer with recurrent bacterial vaginosis to take vitamin D regularly and guess what? It goes away. The other thing is, look at African American women, especially in the North. They have a higher incidence of bacterial vaginosis, and guess what? They are prone to lower vitamin D levels because they have darker skin.

And what's interesting is in the dairy industry, there has been some work looking at giving cows vitamin D by injecting it into their udders to reduce the risk of mastitis. So, vitamin D is really important for bacterial balance and one's own immune system. There is a lot of work being done on vitamin D modulating the immune system. Low vitamin D levels are associated with multiple sclerosis. There is some thought that people are healthier, and have shorter courses of influenza and phenomena, if their vitamin D levels are normal. Vitamin D is there for more than just bones. It is there for immune system health. That's another thing I try to get women to do, when they have what I think is this dysbiosis of this chronic breast pain, I have them take high levels of vitamin D.

BR: What level of vitamin D do you want moms to have?

AE: 50–80.

BR: So that may be something a doctor might consider if a mom is having chronic breast pain . . . and things aren't working to help clear up the pain. They might consider having the mother do a vitamin D test to check her levels.

AE: Low D may not be causative. You still probably have to treat the infection. I still have to get them out of the situation with the biofilm. It doesn't seem to rectify itself. Taking vitamin D is hopefully preventive. I don't know that for sure. Once women have what I believe to be dysbiosis, I can't get it to go away just by having them take high doses of D.

BR: No, I assume an antibiotic of some sort.

AE: Right. Then the other thing is, there has also been some work in Spain looking at Lactobacillus salivarius. You know how we talk about taking probiotics for your gut or for your vagina? Well, the science has now demonstrated that people need to take probiotics that are specific to the issue that they have. And so, for the breast, the specific probiotic is Lactobacillus salivarius. There are some brands of probiotics that have it. So, when I'm treating women, I make sure they are taking that particular type of probiotic. And then an antibiotic, if we have to.

BR: So, the shooting pains that we used to think was ductal yeast, what you are saying (the yeast from the baby's mouth) is triggering the response in the mom's body. It's not yeast at all. It is a type of bacteria, the biofilm.

AE: Yeah. I don't know for sure that everyone has biofilm. I just call it dysbiosis, where things are just out of balance and that causes pain. It's very similar to the symptoms women with bacteria vaginosis experience; they have itchy, burning pain, sometimes sharp shooting pains up through into their uterus.

BR: Very interesting . . . Lisa Amir talks about women who are diagnosed as having a yeast overgrowth . . . that taking a course of Diflucan cures 100% of mothers. By the way, I am not talking about moms that have chronic yeast problems. They fall into a different category. We are talking about mothers who all of sudden do have a yeast overgrowth; a short course of Diflucan should take care of it. So, we have moms who have been boiling pump parts, sterilizing this, sterilizing that, on and off of Diflucan for 6 months.

AE: Exactly. My personal conviction is that Diflucan is antibacterial to some degree. A lot of women who come to see me, they will have been on fluconazole for 7–10 days, or 2 weeks, depending on who gave her the prescription. When asked how much that helped, they say 40%–60%. And what is interesting is 100% of the time, if a mom has only been taking fluconazole, their cultures are negative; they don't have any Staph epi. There has been no research that I can see to show whether or not fluconazole is anti-bacterial. But I suspect it is because these moms should have normal levels of Staph epi. Everyone has it and their cultures are totally sterile. So (the fluconazole) is killing something.

BR: Right. I have also heard that Diflucan, fluconazole, is an anti-inflammatory, which can help you feel better while you are taking it.

AE: Yes. That's true, too.

BR: What are some of the key questions IBCLCs need to ask a mom with nipple pain or breast pain? What questions can we use to pin point are we talking about yeast or are we talking about bacterial? Are we thinking about vasospasm? Are we thinking about latch? Baby damage?

AE: One of the lactation consultant's main roles is to help with latching and positioning. Make sure it's not the most common cause, which is going to be infant positioning and latch. Her role is to ask about the nature of the pain. Does the pain occur with latch? That's a clue. If the pain continues throughout the feeding, that would be consistent with it being a latch-and-suck issue. If the baby latches really well, the nipple is way back by the uvula in the baby's mouth. Women with chronic pain from a dysbiosis are usually not bothered much by pain during the course of the feeding. Sometimes at the end of the feed, they start to get bothered again. If the pain is continuing throughout the feeding, then you really want to think about whether or not it is a latch issue. And of course, watching to see what things look like, to see how the baby nursed. Check to see if there is ongoing nipple trauma, if the nipple looks pinched or distorted. Try to fix positioning, the way she is latching, or the way she is delatching, whatever it is.

If the pain seems to happen after nursing, then I think more about bacterial infection or dysbiosis. Now the trick in between here will be in determining vasospasm. With vasospasm, a lot of time the pain won't start during the course of nursing. It is easy to identify because the nipple will look pale or purple after feeding when the baby comes off. Where it gets messy is if the mom is having vasospasms due to infection. Then someone might have a difficult time sorting out whether the pain is due to vasospasm or infection. The way I sort that out is by asking the mom if she has pain at times the nipple is not pale or purple. If the pain continues to go on for an hour after nursing, but the nipple is only pale or purple for 15 minutes, then I more strongly suspect infection. The moms say they only have pain when the nipple is pain or purple, when they get out of the shower, when they change their shirt. That's when it hurts. The other clue to figure out if vasospasm is due to infection is, does heat help? Because heat by itself is not going to help a chronic dysbiosis type pain. But it's going to help immensely with vasospasm pain. Women will notice right away, "Wow, that really takes the pain away." And then you can better determine what it is. I would say from my experience, it's very uncommon for the pain to be primarily vasospasms. It's probably 5% of the women with chronic pain. I see a lot of women with chronic pain. Probably only 5% are 100% vasospasm.

BR: This is new to me. I did not know a vasospasm could be caused by an infection . . . that it could be a symptom of infection. Can you tell me a little more about that and how that works?

AE: I don't know why it works that way. It can be primary where it is just a vasospasm, or it can be secondary due to trauma and infection. I think that the majority of the cases that I see are due to trauma. And the nipple doesn't progress (to changing colors). It just stays pale, and the pain is not directly associated with the color of the nipple. The mothers won't have pain when the nipple is pale, and they will have pain when the nipple looks normal. The other big reason a nipple can look pale or purple can be due to pumping. Pumping can be pretty traumatic.

BR: Right. Often moms have no idea that different shield sizes exist and that pumps should only be turned up so far.

More pressure or vacuum is not better. There are a lot of bad pumps on the market.

AE: We also need different shaped breast shields. Breasts come in all shapes and sizes.

BR: Often, the IBCLC is the one who is looking at these moms and sorting out what the pain might be from. They have a theory as to the cause of the pain. What are the next steps? Obviously, refer back to the primary healthcare provider, but what does that person do? What do you do?

AE: I do a culture, often a course of antibiotics that that particular bacteria is sensitive to. This can involve long courses of antibiotics. You need a doctor who is willing to try this and check back in 2 weeks to make sure things are working. If things aren't working, you have to try something else. Follow-up is key. You need good enough improvement to stay on that course of antibiotics. It does take a little bit of experience to know how to treat. I think there are a lot of women who never get their pain taken care of.

BR: I do, too. And we know that pain is one of the most common reasons to quit breastfeeding. So, if we can't get that pain resolved for her, the odds of her weaning early are greatly increased. So, it sounds like so much more education needs to be done in the medical community.

AE: Absolutely. And there needs to be a lot more follow-up. That is what concerns me about the tongue-tie clipping. "See ya, come back if there is a problem" is what moms are told after a clipping. A mom is not likely to come back if she is still in pain. You have to schedule them back to follow-up. Follow-up is important because if they don't have the support, they are going to think, "Okay, well, I guess that's it." They don't have any hope that anyone can help them. So, we don't have a lot of good follow-up studies on chronic breast pain. That's why I only give 1–2 weeks of antibiotics at a time. I need my mom to come back and let me know what is going on. I think follow-up is really important.

BR: When IBCLCs and physicians are working with mothers, moms need to hear that this is just a first course of action, and if this does not work, then there are other things to try. Sometimes you don't know what the problem is until you try the treatment, and then if it responds to treatment, and then that can help you make another diagnosis. They need to hear that loud and clear. If this doesn't work, we will try something else.

BR: Thank you so much for taking the time for this interview! Anything else you would like to add?

AE: You're welcome. Let me tell you a little bit more about my latest project, The Milk Mob. The goal of The Milk Mob is to partner with communities and medical systems that want to train their nurses and other outpatient supporters in breastfeeding. We are looking for groups that want outpatient breastfeeding training. If you want more info, go to https://themilkmob.org/ Our first program, The Office Nurse Breastfeeding Champion, is a 16-hour course designed to provide breastfeeding support in the primary care medical home (family physician, pediatrician, midwife, and/or obstetrician's office). This program teaches office nurses, medical assistants, and other outpatient health professional's practical and evidence-based breastfeeding triage and management skills.

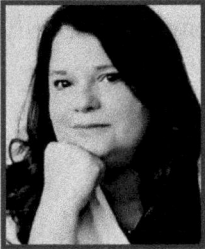

Barbara D. Robertson, IBCLC, has been involved in education for more than 28 years. She received a bachelor's degree in Elementary Education in 1988 and her master's in Education in 1995. Barbara left teaching elementary students in 1995 to raise her two children. Barbara is now the director of The Breastfeeding Center of Ann Arbor. Barbara has developed a 90-hour professional lactation training, a 20-hour course which fulfills the "Baby Friendly" education requirements, and is a speaker for hire on a wide variety of topics including motivational interviewing. Barbara volunteered for the United States Lactation Consultation Association (USLCA) as the director of Professional Development for 4.5 years. She is currently an associate editor for Clinical Lactation, a journal she helped create for USLCA. Barbara has free podcasts, a blog, and YouTube videos, which can all be found on her website http://bfcaa.com/. She has written many articles and created a phone app for working and breastfeeding mothers. She loves working with mothers and babies, helping them with breastfeeding problems in whatever way she can.

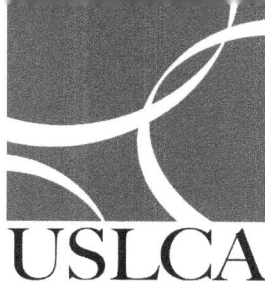

IBCLCs and Craniosacral Therapists

Strange Bedfellows or a Perfect Match?

Patricia Berg-Drazin, IBCLC, RLC, CST

Keywords: ankyloglossia, tongue-tie, lactation, breastfeeding, craniosacral therapy

The rate of ankyloglossia (tongue-tie) appears to be on the rise in the United States and around the world. IBCLCs working with the families of babies with tongue-tie all too often are the first ones to notice the symptoms and suggest treatment. Even after the tongue has been released, these infants continue to struggle with breastfeeding. The tongue plays an integral role in breastfeeding, but it is also crucial to other oral functions such as speech, respiration, oral hygiene, swallowing, and chewing. The tongue is connected through the extrinsic muscles to bone both above and below the oral cavity. The restriction of the tongue results in associated strains in the body. We will follow the muscular connections and origins to understand the influences in the body. Cranio-

sacral therapy (CST) has its origin in osteopathy, which teaches that structure and function are reciprocally interrelated. When structure is compromised, function will be as well. CST is a perfect complement to help these infants' bodies release the tensions created as well as to aid in rebalancing structurally and somatically. A case study will illuminate the tremendous impact CST can have on children suffering from tongue-tie.

Health organizations worldwide unanimously agree that breastfeeding is the best source of nutrition for the optimal health, development, and growth of an infant (Academy of Breastfeeding Medicine, 2008; American Academy of Family Physicians, 2012; American Academy of Pediatrics, 2012; United Nations Children's Emergency Fund, 2014; World Health Organization, 2015). They all recommend breastmilk as the sole source of nutrition for the first 6 months of life.

Ankyloglossia, more commonly known as tongue-tie, can cause breastfeeding difficulties or a cessation of breast-feeding. Mothers of babies with ankyloglossia experience similar difficulties as mothers who wean prematurely. These difficulties include, but are not limited to, sore, cracked, and/or bleeding nipples; engorgement; recurrent plugged ducts; mastitis; breast abscess; poor milk supply; an unsettled baby; frequent feeds; and faltering growth (Ballard, Auer, & Khoury, 2002; Buryk, Bloom, & Shope, 2011; Fernando, 1998; Finigan & Long, 2013; Geddes et al., 2008; Griffiths, 2004; Masaitis & Kaempf, 1996; McAndrew et al., 2012; Messner, Lalakea, Aby, Macmahon, & Bair, 2000; Praborini, Purnamasari, Munandar, & Wulandari, 2015; Ricke, Baker, Madlon-Kay, & DeFor, 2005; Todd, 2014; Todd & Hogan, 2015). It has been reported that ankyloglossia has resulted in babies consuming insufficient breastmilk resulting in failure to thrive (Ballard et al., 2002; Forlenza, Black, McNamara, & Sullivan, 2010; A. Velasco, personal communication, May 7, 2014).

The diminished range of motion stemming from tongue-tie has been implicated in dysfunctions ranging from a higharched palate, problems with swallowing, malocclusion, articulation in speech, oral motor dysfunctions, oral–facial structure mobility, uncontrollable salivation, and an inability to perform dental hygiene later on in life (Cockley & Lehman, 2015; Defabianis, 2000; Fernando, 1998; Haham, Marom, Mangel, Botzer, & Dolberg, 2014; Hall & Renfrew, 2005; Hazelbaker, 2010; Kupietzky & Botzer, 2005; Medeiros, Ferreira, & Felicio, 2009; Meenakshi & Jagannathan, 2014; Praborini et al., 2015; Walls et al., 2014; Watson-Genna, 2013).

There is muscular tension that accompanies tongue-tie, which is frequently not released when the tongue-tie is revised. Infants experiencing feeding difficulties may become stressed. The sympathetic nervous system can go into overdrive (Fernando, 1998). Professional experience and shared cases suggest that craniosacral therapy (CST) can be effective in both releasing the tension that remains after the tongue-tie is released as well, restoring the central nervous system to optimal performance (Jones & Prasaka, 2014; Kotlow, 2015; Wanveer, 2009).

Tongue-tie and the treatment thereof are not a new phenomenon.

In the King James Version Bible–Mark 7:35:

A child's being tongue-tied will impede and hinder his sucking freely. When that happens, he may be observed to lose his hold very often, and, when he draws the breast he frequently makes a clicking noise. Upon this occasion the mouth must be examined and the tongue set at liberty by cutting a ligament or string which will be found to confine the tongue down to the lower part of the mouth.

Statistically speaking, the occurrence of tongue-tie appears to be increasing. In a 1941 study, it was found that 4 in 1,000 infants suffered from ankyloglossia (Fernando, 2015). Studies done between 2000 and 2005 found a range of 3.2%–12.8% of newborns were tongue-tied (Ballard et al., 2002; Dollberg, Marom, & Botzer, 2014; Messner et al., 2000; Praborini et al., 2015; Ricke et al., 2005).

In reality, the rate of occurrence is most likely considerably higher. There is no agreed upon qualitative tool for tongue-tie evaluation. This was demonstrated by Haham et al. (2004) who found that in 200 infants, all but one had either an observable or palpable lingual frenulum using the Coryllos classification (Coryllos, Watson-Genna, & Salloum, 2004). Infants upon birth are not routinely checked for tongue-tie. The Assessment Tool for Lingual Frenulum Function (ATLFF; Hazelbaker, 1993) is the most commonly used evaluation method. Concern has been expressed that the ATLFF contains too many subjective components and lacks inter-rater reliability (McAndrew et al., 2012; Ricke et al., 2005; Rowan-Legg, 2015). Ballard et al. (2002) discloses that the ATLFF has not been validated in a controlled manner.

The Tongue and Its Connections

Ankyloglossia comes from the Greek words agkilos for crooked or loop and glossa for tongue. The frenulum under the tongue is tethering the tongue to the floor of the mouth. This "tether" restricts the tongue's range of motion and, by extension, restricts the motion of every other muscle or bone that it is attached to. To better understand the etiology of these restrictions, we need to start with an understanding of the anatomy of the tongue and how the tongue relates to the rest of the body.

The tongue is made up of intrinsic and extrinsic muscles. The intrinsic muscles have both their origin and their insertion within the tongue. The extrinsic muscles originate in bones and insert in the tongue. The extrinsic muscles are anchored to bones. We want to look more closely at the extrinsic muscles and follow their paths to understand the strain patterns created.

The extrinsic muscles are the genioglossi, geniohyoid, hyoglossi, styloglossi, and the mylohyoid (Figures 1 and 2; Table 1).

One additional muscle of importance to us is the palatoglossus. The palatoglossus muscle forms the anterior portion of the arch from which the uvula hangs. From the undersurface of the soft palate, the palatoglossus curves downward and inserts into the side of the tongue. Tension on this muscle created by a tongue-tie may be a contributory factor in the high palate often seen with tongue-tied individuals (Figure 2; Table 1).

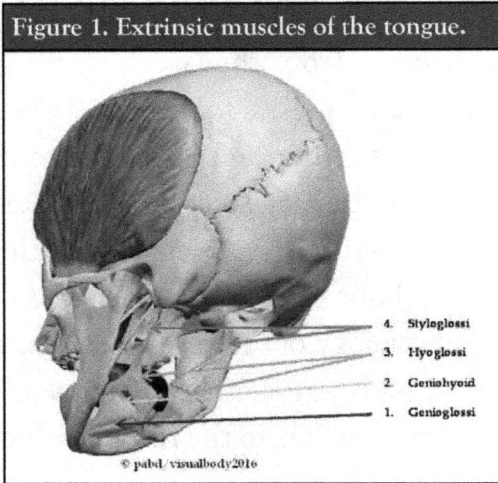

Figure 1. Extrinsic muscles of the tongue.

4. Styloglossi
3. Hyoglossi
2. Geniohyoid
1. Genioglossi

© pabd/visualbody2016

Note. Photo used with permission.

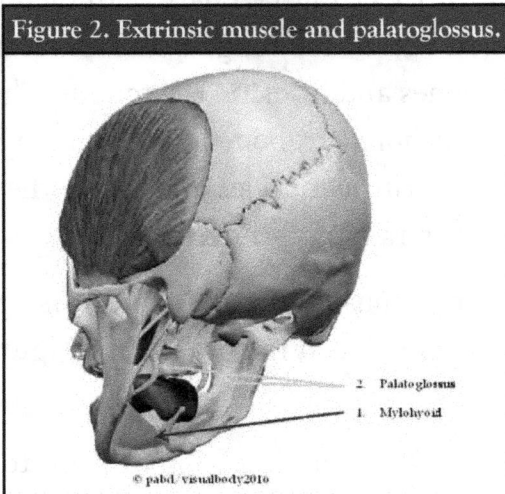

Figure 2. Extrinsic muscle and palatoglossus.

2. Palatoglossus
1. Mylohyoid

© pabd/visualbody2016

Note. Photo used with permission.

Table 1. Figures 1 and 2			
Muscle	Origin	Insertion	Figure
Genioglossi	Mental spine of the mandible	Length of the tongue	1-1
Geniohyoid	Mental spine of the mandible	Superior body of the hyoid	1-2
Hyoglossi	Greater horn of the hyoid	Lateral surface of the tongue	1-3
Styloglossi	Anterior and lateral surface of the styloid process near its apex	Lateral surface of the tongue	1-4
Mylohyoid	Mandible	Hyoid	2-1
Palatoglossus	Palatine aponeurosis	Posterolateral tongue	2-2

There are some common areas of tension seen in babies with ankyloglossia that may be explained by looking at this musculature.

The mandible of a baby with ankyloglossia maybe retracted more than "normal" for a newborn—the genioglossus and geniohyoid originating from the inside surface of the mandible and inserting along the entire length of the tongue could pull the mandible posteriorly (toward the back). The retraction of the mandible can impede effective milk transfer (see Figure 6; Watson Genna, 2013).The styloglossi attaches to the styloid process, the styloid process attaches to the temporalis. When the tongue is tethered, the styloglossi will be pulled anteriorly (forward) and inferiorly (downward). This may put tension on the cranium, starting at the styloid process, and may affect the temporal, parietal, and occipital bones. This tension could be the cause of the chronic headaches that tongue-tied adults have shared experiencing. They often resolve after tongue-tie revision. Infants, if they are having headaches, are unable to communicate that to us.

Infants are unable to communicate what hurts, therefore listening to adults sharing their experiences pre- and post-revision gives us insight into what infants may be experiencing. Adults have spoken of the elimination of headaches, experiencing greater ability to open their mouths and improved speech. One woman shared that her hip alignment improved (Fetzik, 2014; Morgan, n.d.). Another woman shared her difficulty swallowing prerevision and its improvement after (L. Anderegg, personal communication, October 29, 2014). Recently, several adults, in an adult tongue-tie group, have shared structural changes and greater height measurements post-tongue-tie revision. This would follow the strains discussed on the sternum (Figures 3 and 4).

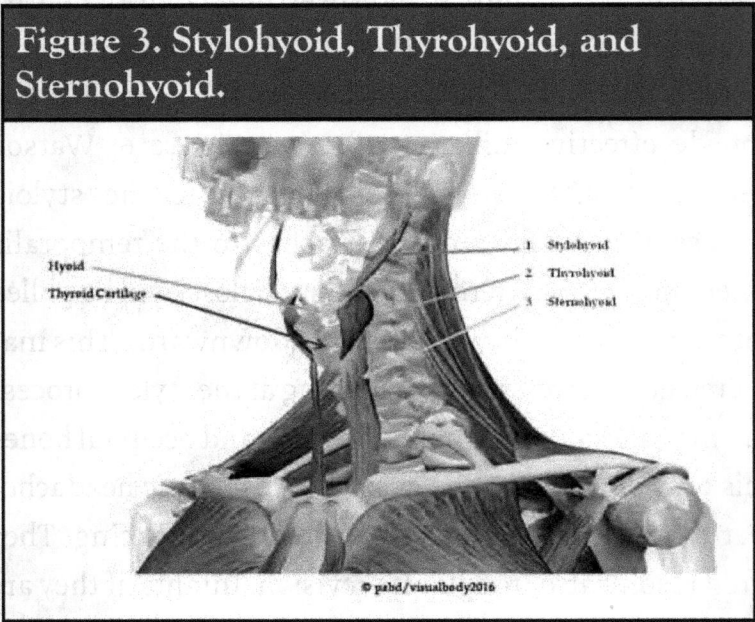

Figure 3. Stylohyoid, Thyrohyoid, and Sternohyoid.

Note. Photo used with permission.

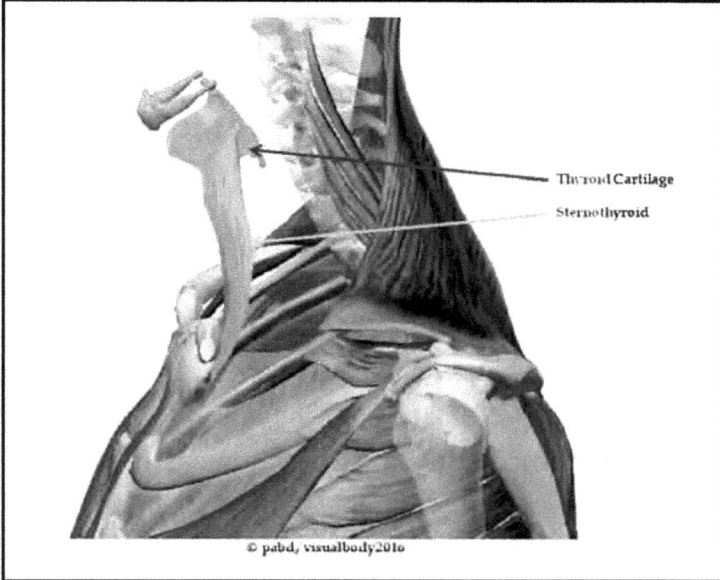

Figure 4. Sternothyroid.

Thyroid Cartilage

Sternothyroid

© pabd, visualbody2016

Note. Photo used with permission.

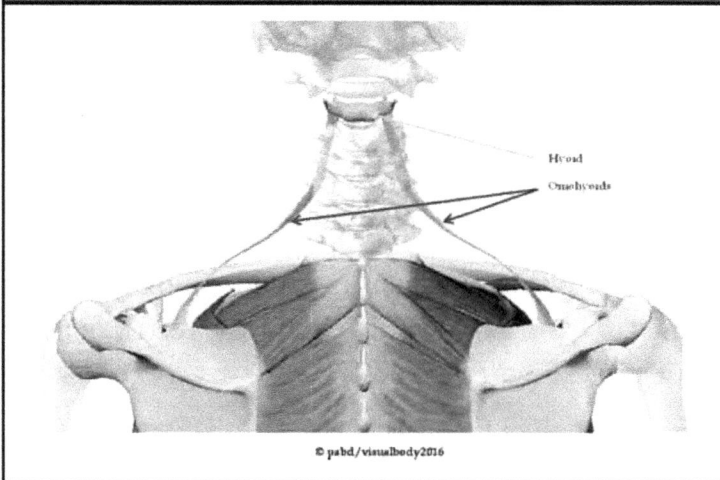

Figure 5. Omohyoid.

Hyoid

Omohyoids

© pabd/visualbody2016

Note. Photo used with permission.

The palatoglossus pulling down on the palatines could explain the higher palates that are often seen in tongue-tied infants and adults. Defabianis (2000) published a case report in which, following the revision of the tongue, there was spontaneous expansion of the upper arch. The patient was followed clinically and radiologically for 7 years (Figure 2).

Neck and sternum tension seen in tongue-tied babies follow the restrictions created by the genioglossi, geniohyoid, and hyoglossi on the hyoid. The hyoid bone connects the floor of the oral cavity to the pharynx and larynx. The genioglossi, geniohyoid, and the hyoglossi all attach to the hyoid. If the tongue has no motion, the hyoid will be tethered, as will all of its attachments (Figure 3; Table 1).

The next step in this process is to look at the muscles that attach to the hyoid and trace them. These are the stylohyoid, thyrohyoid, sternohyoids, sternothyroid, and omohyoids (Figures 3, 4 and 5; Table 2).

Structural observations of infants at rest with ankyloglossia include thoracic tension, raised arms, and hips in flexion (see below). Osteopathy teaches that structure and function are reciprocally interrelated. When structure is compromised, function is compromised (see Figures 6–8).

Following the musculature and looking at the infant depicted in Figure 7, you can see how the restrictions of the tongue travel down the body.

The stylohyoid pulls from the styloid process to the hyoid, the sternohyoids pulls from the hyoid to the sternum (Figures 3 and 4).

The thyrohyoid pulls from the hyoid to the thyroid cartilage, the sternothyroid pulls from the thyroid cartilage to the sternum (Figure 3; Table 2).

The omohyoids are pulling on the scapula. The arm raising may help relieve some of the tension created by the omohyoids. (Figure 5; Table 2).

Releasing the restriction on the tongue does not necessarily translate to the other muscles that are holding tension. Both the neural and the muscular components need to be educated into correct firing and movement patterns. This is where CST can be advantageous.

What Is Craniosacral Therapy?

CST has its origin in osteopathic medicine. It started with Andrew Still. As was common in the 1890s, Andrew apprenticed with his father, a physician, and followed in his father's footsteps. Andrew lost his first wife, Mary, to childbirth complications. Not long after, he lost three of his children to meningitis, despite the fact that they received the standard care of those times. Andrew's daughter by his second wife died of pneumonia. Andrew attributed these deaths to the medical practices of the day. This led him to look for alternative ways of treating disease. He investigated hydropathy, diet, bonesetting, homeopathy, and magnetic healing in his search for a way to enhance nature's own healing abilities.

Table 2. Figures 3, 4, and 5			
Muscle	Origin	Insertion	Figure
Stylohyoid	Stylo process	Hyoid	3-1
Thyrohyoid	Thyroid cartilage	Hyoid	3-2
Sternohyoid	Sternum	Hyoid	3-3
Sternothyroid	Sternum	Thyroid cartilage	4-1
Omohyoid	Scapula	Hyoid	5-1

He believed that "rational medical therapy" would one day consist of manipulations of the musculoskeletal system. The key was to find and correct anatomical deviations that interfered with the free flow of the blood and nerve force in the body. To that end, he developed osteopathy and opened the first osteopathic school in 1892.

William Sutherland was a student of Dr. Still. Dr. Still encouraged students to further his explorations and to "keep digging." Dr. Sutherland was the first person to perceive the movements of the cranial bones. He developed the concept of "primary respiration" to describe the motion created by the cerebral spinal fluid. Dr. Sutherland developed "cranial osteopathy."

John Upledger, DO, FAAO, took the next step. Dr. Upledger, along with a neurophysiologist and histologist, Ernest W. Retzlaff, researched Dr. Sutherland's theory of cranial motion and primary respiration. Their published results supported Dr. Sutherland's theories. Dr. Upledger opened his institute to educate the public and healthcare professionals about the benefits of CST. Dr. Upledger explains CST as "a gentle, hands-on method of evaluating and enhancing the function of the physiological body system called the craniosacral system—compromised of the membranes and the cerebrospinal fluid that surround and protect the brain and the spinal cord. Using a soft touch, generally no greater than 5 grams, or about the weight of a nickel, practitioners release restrictions in the craniosacral system and thereby improve the functioning of the central nervous system. By complementing the body's natural healing processes, CST is increasingly used as a preventative healthcare measure for its ability to bolster resistance to disease, and is effective for a wide range of medical problems associated with pain and dysfunction (The Upledger Institute, 2011).

Craniosacral Therapy for the Baby With Ankyloglossia

Using the craniosacral system's motion, the craniosacral therapist can locate areas that are restricted and/or unbalanced because of the strain on the system from the restriction of the tongue. Using very light touch, between zero to one gram for an infant, the craniosacral therapist assists the body in gaining its full range of motion. The body needs a full range of motion for optimal functioning.

CST also helps to balance and give flexibility to the nervous system. The nervous system is made up of the sympathetic and the parasympathetic nervous systems. The sympathetic nervous system responds to danger, whereas the parasympathetic monitors bodily functions. There are stressors in all of our lives on a regular basis. The sympathetic nervous system is activated with each of these occurrences. Sometimes, the body has difficulty dispersing the accumulated stress. CST can help to restore the nervous system and give it flexibility in order for the system to respond more effectively to stresses and challenges.

Babies go through many transitions that can be extremely stressful in a very short time span. Some manage these transitions (stressors) better than others. After birth, infants have to learn to manage all of the functions that previously have been taken care of for them. Difficulties with sucking, swallowing, breathing, and eating create additional unexpected stressors.

The releasing of the tongue-tie will not necessarily release the musculature that has been restricted because of the tongue-tie. The musculature often needs assistance to know that it is now safe to let go and learn to move as the body intends. The sympathetic nervous system needs assistance dispersing the accumulated stress. This is where CST can play an important role.

Case Study

Baby Jane (fictional name) was born by cesarean section because of a breach presentation. The mother reported that Jane was latching on within an hour of delivery and appeared to be breastfeeding well during their 4-day hospital stay. On Day 5, mother and baby saw their pediatrician who made no mention of a lip or tongue-tie.

They had an IBCLC come to their home the following week because mom was struggling with unresolving engorgement. The IBCLC did not do an intraoral assessment of the infant but told her "everything looked good."

After another week, Mom's engorgement progressively got worse, and Jane was having difficulty feeding. The IBCLC returned and this time did a before-and-after-feeding weighing. Three ounces were transferred in one feeding. The IBCLC looked in Jane's mouth and noticed a tongue-tie.

With Jane's increasing fussiness and difficulty feeding, Mom took Jane to another pediatrician who noted a liptie and recommended a local dentist who does lip and tongue-tie revisions.

The dentist saw Jane that afternoon. He also noted that there was a tongue-tie. Both were revised. Both were considered Class 3 using the Coryllos/Watson Genna classification (Coryllos et al., 2004).

Post-revision, the dentist, on hearing her list of difficulties, recommended that Mom take Jane to a CST to help work though some of the restrictions and stresses that would remain despite the revision.

Jane saw the craniosacral therapist 24 hours post-revision. Both parents went to the session. They shared with the craniosacral therapist, prior to the session, that Jane was so "tight" that Mom was unable to hold and comfort her. She was constantly fussy, which was making parenting and breastfeeding difficult. Mom also noticed that Jane preferred laying her head to one side as shown in Figure 8. The omohyoids originate in the scapula and insert into the hyoid. The hyoid is restricted by the tongue-tie. The infant raises her arms to reduce the strain from the tension of the omohyoids (Figures 5 and 8; Table 2).

Some craniosacral therapists start by placing babies on a blanket and sharing with the parents a structural assessment. As seen earlier, the arms are raised, the head turns left—parents may not notice these things or be aware that they are indications of restrictions and tension (Simpson, 2015).

Babies are usually treated on a blanket or on the therapist's lap. Infant sessions are generally an hour in length. Breaks are taken as needed for feeding and changing.

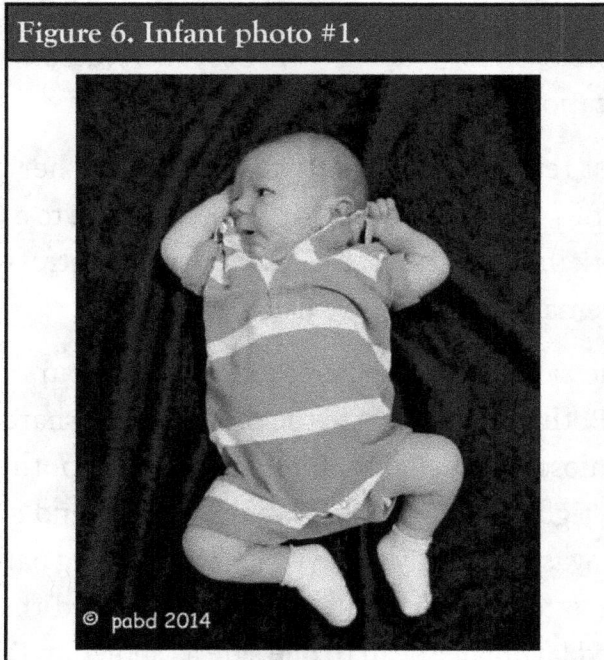

Figure 6. Infant photo #1.

© pabd 2014

Note. Photo used with permission.

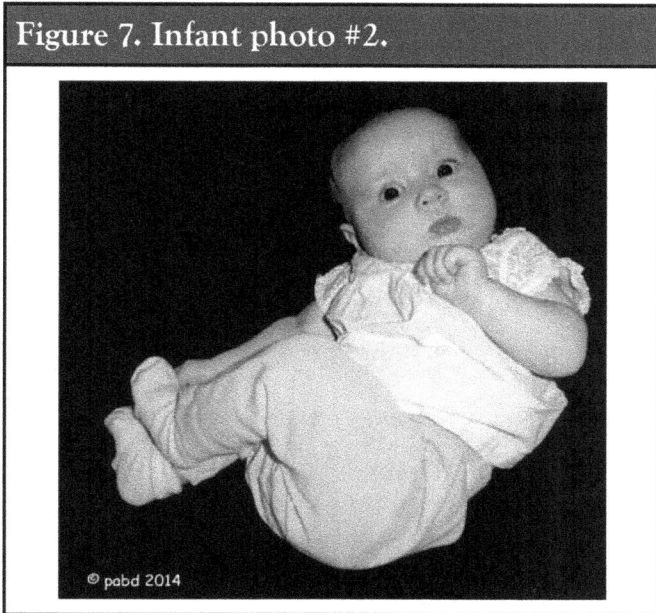

Figure 7. Infant photo #2.

© pabd 2014

Note. Photo used with permission.

There were significant restrictions in the thoracic area, as well as across the scapula. When you follow the pathway from the tongue, as discussed earlier, the restriction in the scapula and thoracic area is understandable. There may be other patterns of restriction as well.

When Jane was handed back to her mother post therapy session, Jane "melted" into Mom's chest. Both parents started to cry. Jane's mother said that this was the first time Jane had melted into her and that she had been able to hold her.

Upon follow-up, Mom shared that,

> when we came home from the craniosacral therapy, things were amazing. Jane was so calm and seemed so happy.

It took about 3 days, but she was able to eat on either breast and in whatever position we wanted. We were normally doing cradle before the pulling away from the breast started to happen. [After the treatment], Jane was doing great; she was far less fussier and was sleeping better at night, too. She also wasn't clenching her arms above her head as much. I [mom] noticed she wasn't always putting her head to the right all the time.

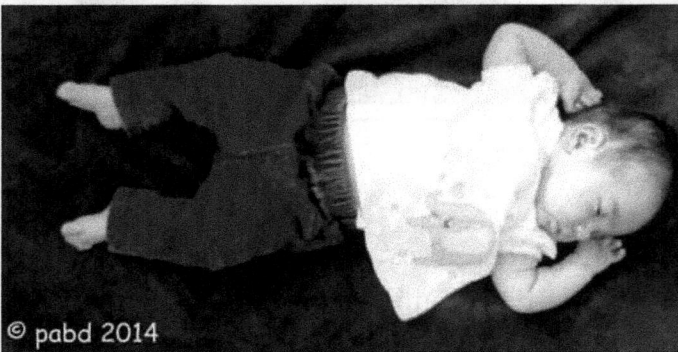

Figure 8. Infant photo #3.

© pabd 2014

Note. Photo used with permission.

These are tremendous results following one craniosacral session. One cannot expect all babies to experience such an incredible response. It is the author's experience that tremendous results appear to be commonplace following either one or several treatments.

Discussion

The African proverb attributed to Margaret Mead, "it takes a village to raise a child," also should apply to healthcare professionals of different disciplines working together sharing knowledge and skills for the betterment of the child and the family.

The IBCLC assisting struggling new parents are often the first to notice the tongue's restrictions. Parents may then be referred to local dentists; ear, nose, and throat specialists; or other medical professionals who have an understanding of ankyloglossia and are trained in revision (Ballard et al., 2002; Fernando, 1998; Finigan & Long, 2013; Watson Genna, 2002). On recommendation of the lactation consultant or the provider who will be doing the revision, many parents are referred to a craniosacral therapist prior to having the revision done and again after the procedure. We are the village—the IBCLC who helps to uncover the cause of the difficulty, the practitioner who revises, and the craniosacral therapist who, with an understanding that structure and function are reciprocally interrelated, can help the infant's body regain its optimal structure and fluidity of movement. We need to work in concert to raise the next generation so that they can rise to their highest potential.

References

Academy of Breastfeeding Medicine. (2008). ABM statement: Position on breastfeeding. *Breastfeeding Medicine, 3*(4), 267–270.

American Academy of Family Physicians. (2012). *Breastfeeding (policy statement)*. Retrieved from http://www.aafp.org/about/policies/all/breastfeeding.html

American Academy of Pediatrics. (2012). Policy statement: Breastfeeding and the use of human milk. *Pediatrics, 129,* e827–e841.

Ballard, J. L., Auer, C. E. D., & Khoury, J. C. (2002). Ankyloglossia: Assessment, incidence, and effect of frenuloplasty on the breastfeeding dyad. *Pediatrics, 110*(5), e63. Retrieved from http://www.pediatrics.org/cgi/content/110/5/e63

Buryk, M., Bloom, D., & Shope, T. (2011). Efficacy of neonatal release of ankyloglossia: A randomized trial. *Pediatrics, 128*(2), 280–288.

Cockley, L., & Lehman, A. (2015). The ORTHO missing link: Could it be tied to the tongue? *Journal of the American Orthodontic Society, 15*(1), 18–21.

Coryllos, E., Watson Genna, C., & Salloum, A. (2004). *Congenital tongue-tie and its impact on breastfeeding.* Elk Grove Village, IL: American Academy of Pediatrics, Section on Breastfeeding.

Defabianis, P. (2000). Ankyloglossia and its influence on maxillary and mandibular development (A seven-year follow-up case report). *The Functional Orthodontist, 17*(4), 25–33.

Dollberg, S., Marom, R., & Botzer, E. (2014). Lingual frenotomy for breastfeeding difficulties: A prospective follow-up study. *Breastfeeding Medicine, 9*(6), 286–289.

Fernando, C. (1998). Tongue tie —from confusions to clarity: *A guide to the diagnosis and treatment of ankyloglossia.* Sydney, Australia: Tandem.

Fernando, C. (2015). Tongue tie: *Information for parents and practitioners.* Retrieved from Tonguetie.net

Fetzik, M. (2014). *Celebrating two years migraine free.* Retrieved from http://www.happykansasfaces.com/blog/archives/09-2014

Finigan, V., & Long, T. (2013). The effectiveness of frenulotomy on infant-feeding outcomes: A systematic review. *Evidence Based Midwifery, 11*(2), 40–45.

Forlenza, G., Black, N., McNamara, E., & Sullivan, S. (2010). Ankyloglossia, exclusive breastfeeding, and failure to thrive. *Pediatrics, 125*(6), e1500–1504. Retrieved from http://pediatrics.aappublications.org/content/125/6/e1500

Geddes, D., Langton, D., Gollow, I., Jacobs, L. A., Hartmann, P., & Simmer, K. (2008). Frenulotomy for breasfeeding infants with ankyloglossia: Effect on milk removal and sucking mechanism as imagined by ultrasound. *Pediatrics, 122*(1), e188–194. Retrieved from http://pediatrics.aappublications.org/content/122/1/e188?sso=1&sso_redirect_count=1&nfstatus=401&nftoken=00000000-0000-0000-0000-000000000000&nfstatusdescription=ERROR%3a+No+local+token

Griffiths, D. M. (2004). Do tongue ties affect breastfeeding? *Journal of Human Lactation, 20*(4), 409–414.

Haham, A., Marom, R., Mangel, L., Botzer, E., & Dollberg, S. (2014). Prevalence of breastfeeding difficulties in newborns with a lingual frenulum: A prospective cohort series. *Breastfeeding Medicine, 9*(9), 438–441.

Hall, D. M., & Renfrew, M. J. (2005). Tongue tie. *Archives of Disease in Childhood, 90*, 1211–1215.

Hazelbaker, A. K. (1993). *The assessment tool for lingual frenulum function (ATLFF): Use in a lactation consultant private practice (Master's thesis).* Pacific Oaks College, Pasadena, CA.

Hazelbaker, A. K. (2010). *Tongue-tie: Morphogenesis, impact, assessment and treatment.* Columbus, OH: Aidan and Eva.

Jones, M., & Prasaka, E. (2014). *Manual therapy prior to & after release of tethered oral tissues (commonly called tongue and lip ties).* Retrieved from http://www.musclesinharmony.com/manual-therapy-postrevisions.html

Kotlow, L. (2015). TOTS—tethered oral tissues: The assessment and diagnosis of the tongue and upper lip ties in breastfeeding. *Oral Health*, 64–70.

Kupietzky, A., & Botzer, E. (2005). Ankyloglossia in the infant and young child: Clinical suggestions for diagnosis and management. *Pediatric Dentistry, 27*, 40–46.

Masaitis, N., & Kaempf, J. (1996). Developing a frenotomy policy at one medical center: A case study approach. *Journal of Human Lactation, 12*(3), 229–232.

McAndrew, F., Thompson, J., Fellows, L., Large, A., Speed, M., & Renfrew, M. (2012). *Infant feeding survey 2010: Summary.* Retrieved from hscic.gov.uk/catalogue/PUB08694

Medeiros, A., Ferreira, J., & Felício, C. (2009). Correlations between feeding methods, non-nutritive sucking and orofacial behaviors. *Pro-Fono, 21*(4), 315–319.

Meenakshi, S., & Jagannathan, N. (2014). Assessment of lingual frenulum lengths in skeletal malocclusion. *Journal of Clinical and Diagnostic Research, 8*(3), 202–204.

Messner, A. H., Lalakea, M. L., Aby, J., Macmahon, J., & Bair, E. (2000). Ankyloglossia: Incidence and associated feeding difficulties. *Archives of Otolaryngology–Head & Neck Surgery, 126*(1), 36–39.

Morgan, B. (n.d.) *What we have learned from our tongue tied babies.* Retrieved from http://www.mobimotherhood.org/what-wehave-learned-from-our-tongue-tied-babies.html

Moss, W. (1794). *An essay on the management, nursing and diseases of children from the birth: and on the treatment of diseases of pregnant and lying-in women: With remarks on domestic practice of medicine* (2nd ed.). Egham, United Kingdom: Boult & Longman.

Praborini, A., Purnamasari, H., Munandar, A., & Wulandari, R. (2015). Early frenotomy improves breastfeeding outcomes for tongue-tied infants. *Clinical Lactation, 6*(1), 9–14.

Ricke, L., Baker, N., Madlon-Kay, D., & DeFor, T. (2005). Newborn tongue-tie: Prevalence and effect on breast-feeding. *The Journal of the American Board of Family Practice, 18*(1), 1–7.

Rowan-Legg, A. (2015). Ankyloglossia and breastfeeding. *Paediatrics & Child Health, 20*(4), 209–218.

Simpson, J. (2015). *Structure and function.* http://www.jayesimpson.com/structure-and-function/

Todd, D. (2014). Tongue-tie in the newborn: What, when, who and how? Exploring tongue-tie division. *Breastfeeding Review, 22*(2), 7–10.

Todd, D., & Hogan, M. J. (2015). Tongue-tie in the newborn: Early diagnosis and division prevents poor breastfeeding outcomes. *Breastfeeding Review, 23*(1), 11–16.

United Nations Children's Emergency Fund. (2014). *Infant and young child feeding.* Retrieved from http://www.unicef.org/nutrition/index_breastfeeding.html

The Upledger Institute. (2011). *Discover craniosacral therapy.* Retrieved from www.upledger.com/therapies

Walls, A., Pierce, M., Wang, H., Steehler, A., Steehler, M., & Harley, E., Jr. (2014). Parental perception of speech and tongue mobility in three-year olds after neonatal frenotomy. *International Journal of Pediatric Otorhinolaryngology, 78*, 128–131.

Wanveer, T. (2009, October). The tongue: How craniosacral therapy can help this important muscle. *Massage Magazine.* Retrieved from http://massagemag.com/the-togue-how-craniosacraltherapy-can-help-this-important-muscle-6274/

Watson Genna, C. (2002). Tongue-tie and breastfeeding. *Leaven, 38*(2), 27–29.

Watson Genna, C. (2013). *Supporting sucking skills in breastfeeding infants* (2nd ed.). Burlington, MA: Jones and Bartlett.

World Health Organization. (2015). *Infant and young child feeding.* Retrieved from http://www.who.int/mediacentre/factsheets/fs342/en/

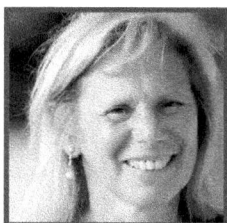

Patricia Berg-Drazin is an Internationally Board Certified Lactation Consultant and a Certified CranioSacral Therapist, who provides a holistic approach to working with her patients. She received her IBCLC certification in 1990. She started studying with the Upledger Institute in 1997 and received her CranioSacral certification in 2010. Patricia sees patients primarily through her private practice, as this affords her the most flexibility in optimal care provision. Patricia continually bolsters her knowledge base by attending and presenting at conferences around the world. She presents on topics ranging from engorgement to the etiology of structural issues that affect breastfeeding, as well as the importance of CranioSacral therapy in tongue-tied infants and children with challenges. Patricia has authored a number of works, including: "Taking Nipple Shields out of the Closet," "A Growth on the Nipple?" (a case study of staph infection on the nipple), and "Using a Mirror to Assist with Pumping." Patricia has two children, Michael and Richard.

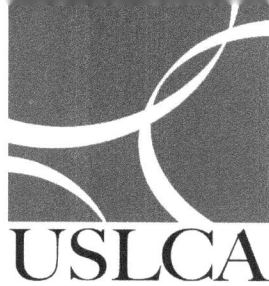

Early Frenotomy Improves Breastfeeding Outcomes for Tongue-Tied Infants

Asti Praborini, MD, IBCLC

Hani Purnamasari, MD

Agusnawati Munandar, MD, IBCLC

Ratih Ayu Wulandari, MD, IBCLC

Keywords: breastfeeding, tongue-tie, frenotomy, lactogenesis

Although there is evidence to suggest that frenotomy improves breastfeeding outcomes for tongue-tied (ankyloglossic) infants, less is known about the optimal timing of treatment. In this retrospective cohort study, the timing of frenotomy and its impact on infant and maternal factors were examined in 31 tongue-tied babies with breastfeeding difficulties in a hospital in Jakarta, Indonesia. After frenotomy, all infants improved latching and mothers experienced a subjective improvement in nipple pain and breast engorgement. Frenotomy improved weight gain in infants regardless of type of tongue-tie (p 5 .001), but greater mean weight gains were achieved in tongue-tied babies who underwent early frenotomy (prior to Day 8) compared to babies who underwent late frenotomy (after Day 8; p 5 0.002). Tongue-tie and frenotomy issues need to be addressed during the very first few days of an infant's life to ensure optimal breastfeeding outcomes.

The International Affiliation of Tongue-tie Professionals defines tongue-tie (ankyloglossia) as "an embryological remnant of tissue in the midline between the undersurface of the tongue and the floor of the mouth that restricts normal tongue movement" (International Affiliation of Tongue-tie Professionals, 2014). The incidence of tongue-tie is reported to be between 1% and 10%, and its association with breastfeeding difficulties is well-documented (Ballard, Auer, & Khoury, 2002; Messner, Lalakea, Aby, Macmahon, & Bair, 2000). These problems include maternal nipple pain, slow infant weight gain, infant breast refusal, and low maternal milk supply because of poor milk removal (Garbin et al., 2013). Frenotomy, in which the lingual frenulum is cut, has been shown to effectively resolve breastfeeding difficulties caused by infants with tongue-tie in several clinical studies (Buryk, Bloom, & Shope, 2011; Geddes et al., 2008; Knox, 2010; Mayer, 2012). However, there have only been limited studies on tongue-tie in Indonesia, and there is little data and no universal guidelines to inform practitioners on the optimal timing of frenotomy (Garbin et al., 2013). There are many videos available online about tongue-tie and breastfeeding: https://www.youtube.com/playlist?list=P-Lae1FWVfiavd8hUop6sSs8Vai68cSYyKD

We therefore examined the effects of early and late frenotomy on breastfeeding outcomes from the perspectives of both the mother and infant. We demonstrate that frenotomy performed as soon as possible, and ideally prior to Day 8, has a greater impact on improving weight gain compared to frenotomy performed after Day 8.

Method

Sample

All pediatric consultation files between January and June 2011 in a hospital with pediatric facilities in South Jakarta, Indonesia, were reviewed. There were 505 patient consultations over the study period, from which 62 tongue-tie cases were identified for an overall incidence of 12.3% in our population; half of these were excluded because of loss to follow-up, leaving 31 cases available for study. Mothers and infants presented with various complaints: Mother complaints included sore nipple(s), breast engorgement, mastitis, pain during breastfeeding, and blocked ducts or nipple pores, whereas infant problems included latching only to the nipple, having a long period of breastfeeding without satiety, rage during breastfeeding, excessive weight loss, or not achieving the recommended weight gain. The subjects' characteristics are shown in Table 1.

A thorough history and examination was performed in all cases, including examination of the mother's breast, breastfeeding dyad, and baby's mouth. Where tongue-tie was found, it was observed to significantly interfere with the breastfeeding dyad. Babies were subsequently grouped according to the Coryllos classification of ankyloglossia, as shown in Table 2 (Genna, 2013).

Table 1. Characteristics of Study Subjects	
Characteristics	N = 31 (%)
Gender	
Male	13 (42%)
Female	18 (58%)
Age	
0–30 days	17 (55%)
1–6 months	14 (45%)
Tongue-tie type	
1	3 (10%)
2	10 (32%)
3	12 (38%)
4	6 (20%)
Age when frenotomy was done	
0–8 days	8 (26%)
>8 days	23 (74%)
Frenotomy indication	
Mother's complain	7 (22%)
Baby's complain	7 (22%)
Mother + baby complain	17 (56%)
Nutritional status	
Failure to thrive	13 (42%)
• An infant with body weight under the 3rd percentile or Z score <-2. This occurred when the infant continued to lose weight after the age of 10 days and did not return to their birth weight by the age of 3 weeks or remained below the 10th percentile by the end of the first month of life.	
Slow weight gain	
• An infant less than 2 weeks of age who is more than 10% less than the birth weight or who is 2 weeks to 3 months of age whose weight gain is less than 20 g/day	10 (32%)
Well growth	
• An infant whose weight increases according to the World Health Organization exclusively breastfed growth curves	8 (26%)

Babies' weights were plotted using the World Health Organization (WHO) Anthro growth and development software. Growth was classified as "good" if the weight increased according to the growth curve (Ng, 2010), whereas weight gain was classified as "slow" if infants less than 2 weeks of age had weight 10% less than the birth weight or infants 2 weeks to 3 months of age gained less than 20 g/day (Walker, 2011a). "Failure to thrive" was defined as body weight under the 3rd percentile or Z score ,2 2, which occurred if the baby continued to lose weight after 10 days and did not return to their birth weight by 3 weeks, or were below the 10th percentile at the end of the first month of life (Ng, 2010).

Table 2. Coryllos Classification of Ankyloglossia			
Type	Superior Attachment	Inferior Attachment	Characteristic of Frenulum
1	Tip of tongue	Alveolar ridge	Often thin, may be elastic
2	2–4 mm behind tongue tip	On or just behind alveolar ridge	Often thin, may be elastic
3	Mid tongue	Middle of floor of mouth	Usually thicker, more fibrous, inelastic
4	Submucosal	Floor of mouth at base of tongue	Usually thick, fibrous, shiny, and inelastic

Source: Genna, C. W. (2013). *Supporting sucking skills in breastfeeding infants.* Sudbury, MA: Jones and Bartlett.

Classification of Frenotomy

Babies were also grouped by the timing of the frenotomy, early and late, which we refer to lactogenesis stage. Lactogenesis Stage II marks the onset of copious milk secretion between Day 3–8; milk synthesis occurs even in the absence of infant suckling or milk expression. Lactogenesis Stage III (Day 9 to the beginning of involution) is the maintenance of established milk production via autocrine control (Riordan, 2010). Although lactogenesis Stages II and III are physiologic processes, and cannot be defined by days of age, for the purposes of this retrospective chart review, we are using days of age as a proxy for stage of lactogenesis, early frenotomy refer to babies who underwent frenotomy in between Day 3 and 8, and late frenotomy refer to babies who underwent frenotomy after Day 9.

Procedure

Parents received a full explanation about tongue-tie and frenotomy and gave written informed consent prior to the procedure. In preparation for frenotomy, the baby was swaddled to immobilize the arms and legs and laid supine on the examination table. An assistant helped by holding the head still while the operator lifted the tongue with a finger to locate the problematic frenulum. The area was disinfected by applying povidone-iodine with swab sticks, as described previously (Sunil Kumar, Raja Babu, Jagadish Reddy, & Uttam, 2011). The frenulum was then snipped with blunt-ended sterile scissors, and sterile gauze was used to attain hemostasis. The tongue-tie was assessed as completely released if a neat diamond shape was visible with no palpable tissue remaining to restrict tongue movement. We favored not using general anesthesia to perform the procedure because this is likely to add delays in breastfeeding.

Immediately after frenotomy, the mother was asked to breastfeed her baby for reevaluation of latch and improvement. The mother was taught how to perform tongue exercises to prevent reattachment, and a review was scheduled 3 days later to assess for complications and evaluate weight gain. A further review was scheduled 1 week later and continued every week thereafter as necessary until the breastfeeding dyads' course was deemed satisfactory.

Data Collection and Analyses

Weight loss data were collected by comparing weight at the time of frenotomy to that infant's birth weight and dividing that by the age of the baby in days on the day of frenotomy. Weight gain data were collected by comparing weight upon the baby review and dividing days on the day of frenotomy. The review time was between 3 days to 1 week after frenotomy.

Standard WHO growth data show that even infants born at and following the 1st percentile gain, at minimum, 30 g/day. However, the WHO system has been shown to result in false positives for the "underweight" category in some breastfed infants during the first 6 months, resulting in unnecessary supplementation or early use of complementary foods (Walker, 2014). Therefore, we regarded a minimum weight gain per day of 20 g to be satisfactory (Ng, 2010).

Data were analyzed using SPSS Version 19. The paired t test was performed to analyze differences in mean weight gain before and after frenotomy. Differences in absolute weight gain before and after frenotomy according to lactogenesis stages were analyzed using the Wilcoxon test.

Results

None of the babies had a good latch prior to frenotomy, in spite of otherwise good breastfeeding positions. Babies nibbled the nipple, made clicking sounds, had dimpled cheeks during breastfeeding, or retracted their lower lip during sucking. After frenotomy, all babies improved their latch. No serious side effects were observed after frenotomy: 6 (20%) babies had minor bleeding that stopped soon after breastfeeding, and at 3 days post-frenotomy, 28 (90%) babies had no observable complications. A white, diamond-shaped wound was observed in three (10%) subjects that disappeared on follow-up a week later. Subjectively, mothers experienced immediate relief after frenotomy, with 27 mothers reporting improvement in nipple pain and breast engorgement after one week, with the remainder improving by two weeks.

The weight loss and gain differences before and after frenotomy for each type of tongue-tie are shown in Table 3. The type of tongue-tie was not associated with weight gain or weight loss. The mean differences in weight loss and weight gain (in grams per day) before and after frenotomy according to type of tongue-tie are shown in Figure 1. Regardless of tongue-tie type, the mean weight loss prior to frenotomy was 18.52 g/day, and the mean weight gain after frenotomy was 27.65 g/day, which was significantly different (p 5 .001). Furthermore, babies lost an average of 65 g/day in weight prior to frenotomy and increased their weight by an average of 38 g/day after frenotomy at lactogenesis Stage II (p 5.002), whereas lactogenesis Stage III babies gained an average of 5 g/day prior to frenotomy but gained 20 g/day after frenotomy, although this change was not statistically significant (p 5 .170; see Figure 2).

Table 3. Weight Loss and Weight Gain Differences Before and After Frenotomy on Each Type of Tongue-Tie				
		Tongue-Tie Type		
Difference in Weight (g/day)	Type 1 (N = 3)	Type 2 (N = 10)	Type 3 (N = 12)	Type 4 (N = 6)
The mean of weight loss before frenotomy	54.78	35.01	4.07	1.81
The mean of weight gain after frenotomy	20.50	32.49	25.72	27.01
Greatest weight loss	35	150	155	33
Greatest weight gain	185	152	45	42

Discussion

Here, we examined the effect of frenotomy on infant weight gain from the perspectives of both the infants and mothers. Frenotomy resulted in significant improvements in weight gain in infants, which was more marked if the frenotomy was performed before Day 8. Since this time point is likely to correspond to lactogenesis Stage II, we hypothesize that optimizing breastfeeding by frenotomy in tongue-tied infants at the same time as the onset of copious milk production contributes to improved early outcomes, at least in terms of weight gain. This finding is in line with a retrospective study by (Steehler, Steehler, & Harley, 2012), who examined data on 367 tongue-tied infants with breastfeeding problems seen over a 5-year period. Based on subjective maternal observations, frenotomy performed on neonates with ankyloglossia and feeding difficulties in the first week of life exhibited more benefit than those who received the procedure after the first week of life.

To ensure successful breastfeeding, health workers who help mothers to breastfeed need to be aware of the complexity and importance of coordinated tongue movements by the infant during feeding. For successful milk extraction, the tongue needs to perform several actions. First, the tongue extends over the lower gum to inhibit the bite reflex and contribute to an airtight seal on the areola to create an intraoral vacuum and promote milk flow from the breast. Second, the tongue needs to manipulate the nipple and areolar tissue into a proper relationship with the hard and soft palates, the tongue itself, and the swallowing/breathing apparatus. Limitation of the tongue's free movement leads to suboptimal nursing mechanics. The nipple's spatial relationship to the infant's mouth structures and the specific pattern of tongue movements are critical both for effective and efficient milk removal and to protect the delicate nipple tissue from trauma. The harmful effects of tongue-tie are either related to ineffective breast emptying, to nipple trauma, or both (Knox, 2010).

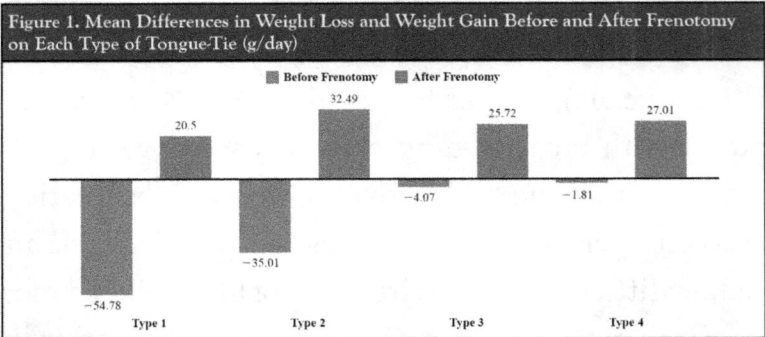

Figure 1. Mean Differences in Weight Loss and Weight Gain Before and After Frenotomy on Each Type of Tongue-Tie (g/day)

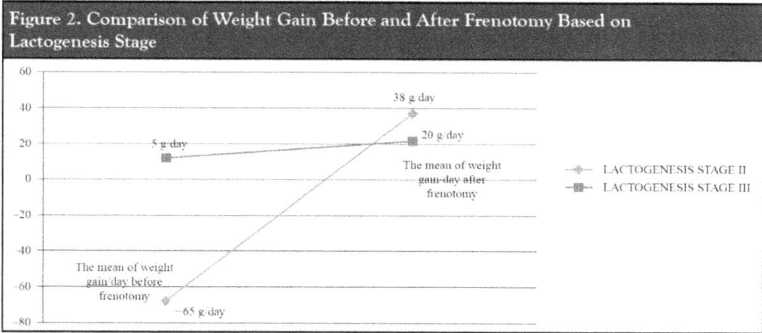

Figure 2. Comparison of Weight Gain Before and After Frenotomy Based on Lactogenesis Stage

Here, we compared two groups: early frenotomy (prior to Day 8 and equivalent to lactogenesis Stage II) and late frenotomy (after Day 8 and equivalent to lactogenesis Stage III).

Lactogenesis refers to the transition from pregnancy to lactation. Lactogenesis Stage I occurs from mid-pregnancy to postpartum Day 2, lactogenesis Stage II from Day 3–8, and lactogenesis Stage III starts on Day 9 and continues to the beginning of involution (Riordan, 2010). After birth, following placental delivery, progesterone levels decline rapidly, resulting in increased prolactin levels and triggering the start of lactogenesis Stage II and the onset of copious milk secretion. Milk synthesis occurs during lactogenesis Stage II even in the absence of infant suckling or milk expression. The volume of milk production increases from 37 ml on Day 1 to 408 ml on Day 3 (the beginning of lactogenesis Stage II), whereas milk volume continues to increase to 576 ml on Day 7 and averages 750 ml by 4 weeks (Walker, 2010b).

Lactogenesis Stage III, also known as galactopoiesis, is the maintenance of the established milk production via autocrine (local) control, in which one type of cell in the gland regulates adjacent cells in the same gland.

Frequent and complete milk removal by feeding is proposed to enhance milk production by removing breast milk constituents that exert negative feedback on breast secretory cells. In this way, removal of milk by the infant controls synthesis and is referred to as the supply-versus-demand response (Black, Jarman, & Simpson, 1998). Although suckling (or mechanical milk removal) may not be a prerequisite for lactogenesis Stage II, it is critical for lactogenesis Stage III. However, the quantity and quality of infant suckling or milk removal governs breast milk synthesis (Riordan, 2010).

Geddes et al. (2008) identified two irregular tongue movements that occur in tongue-tied babies during breastfeeding, which result in compression of the base or the tip of the nipple and may contribute to maternal pain, decreased milk transfer, and consequent slowing weight gain and failure to thrive. Using ultrasound, the same group also showed that frenotomy can resolve irregular tongue movements and improve milk intake, milk transfer rate, attachment to the breast, and maternal pain.

Babies undergoing early frenotomy not only nursed at the breast effectively and efficiently, improving both milk transfer and milk production, but also had sufficient milk volume from intrinsic Stage II milk production to significantly increase weight in these babies. However, late frenotomy (after Day 8), while improving the babies' latch, only resulted in small increases in weight. This is likely to be because of the late release of the tongue-tie creating only a low demand response, leading to low milk transfer and insufficient milk production. Mothers experienced low milk supply, resulting in only small weight gains in these babies who were only breastfed.

Our study was limited by being a retrospective review of medical records, with some records being incomplete. In addition, no control comparison was made with infants not undergoing frenotomy. Further prospective studies with larger sample sizes are required.

Conclusion

For successful lactation, identification of tongue-tie at birth and close monitoring of feeding may help to detect milk supply problems sooner. Frenotomy is an effective, simple, and safe treatment for tongue-tied babies experiencing breastfeeding difficulties. Early frenotomy, prior to Day 8, appears to have a larger impact on weight gain and lactation performance, hence leading to more successful breastfeeding outcomes.

References

Ballard, J. L., Auer, C. E., & Khoury, J. C. (2002). Ankyloglossia: Assessment, incidence, and effect of frenuloplasty on the breastfeeding dyad. *Pediatrics, 110*(5), 63. Retrieved from http://www.pediatrics.org/cgi/content/full/110/5/e63

Black, R. F., Jarman, L., & Simpson, J. B. (1998). *The science of breastfeeding* (Vol. 3). Ontario, Canada: Jones and Bartlett.

Buryk, M., Bloom, D., & Shope, T. (2011). Efficacy of neonatal release of ankyloglossia: A randomized trial. *Pediatrics, 128*(2), 280–288.

Garbin, C. P., Sakalidis, V. S.,Chadwick, L. M., Whan, E., Hartmann, P. E., & Geddes, D. T. (2013). Evidence of improved milk intake after frenotomy: A case report. *Pediatrics, 132*(5), e1413–e1417.

Geddes, D. T., Langton, D. B., Gollow, I., Jacobs, L. A., Hartmann P. E., & Simmer, K. (2008). Frenulotomy for breastfeeding infants with ankyloglossia: Effect on milk removal and sucking mechanism as imaged by ultrasound. *Pediatrics, 122*, e188–e194.

Genna, C. W. (2013). *Supporting sucking skills in breastfeeding infants.* Sudbury, MA: Jones and Bartlett.

International Affiliation of Tongue-tie Professionals. (2014). *Definition of tongue-tie.* Retrieved from http://tonguetieprofessionals.org/about/assessment/definition-of-tongue-tie/

Knox, I. (2010). Tongue tie and frenotomy in the breastfeeding newborn. *Neoreviews, 11*(9), e513–e519. Retrieved from http://neoreviews.aappublications.org/content/11/9/e513.short

Mayer, D. R. (2012, January 1). Frenotomy for breastfed tongue-tied infants: A fresh look at an old procedure. *AAP News, 33*, 12.

Messner, A. H., Lalakea, M. L., Aby, J., Macmahon, J., & Bair, E. (2000). Ankyloglossia: Incidence and associated feeding difficulties. *Archives of Otolaryngology—Head and Neck Surgery, 126*(1), 36–39.

Ng, P. (2010). Low intake in the breastfeeding infant: Maternal and infant considerations. In J. Riordan & K. Wambach (Eds.), *Breastfeeding and human lactation* (4th ed., pp. 325–363). Sudbury, MA: Jones and Bartlett.

Riordan, J. (2010). Anatomical and biological imperatives. In J. Riordan & K. Wambach (Eds.), *Breastfeeding and human lactation* (4th ed., pp. 77–112). Sudbury, MA: Jones and Bartlett.

Steehler, M. W., Steehler, M. K., & Harley, E. H. (2012). A retrospective review of frenotomy in neonates and infants with feeding difficulties. *International Journal of Pediatric Otorhinolaryngology, 76*(9), 1236–1240.

Sunil Kumar, P., Raja Babu, P., Jagadish Reddy, G., & Uttam, A. (2011). Povidone iodine—Revisited. *Indian Journal of Dental Advancements, 3*(3), 617–620.

Walker, M. (2011a). Beyond the initial 48–72 hours: Infant challenges. In *Breastfeeding management for the clinician: Using the evidence* (2nd ed., pp. 347–427). Sudbury, MA: Jones and Bartlett.

Walker, M. (2011b). Influence of the maternal anatomy and physiology. In *Breastfeeding management for the clinician: Using the evidence* (2nd ed., pp. 75–131). Sudbury, MA: Jones and Bartlett.

Walker, M. (2014). Beyond the initial 48–72 hours: *Infant challenges. In Breastfeeding management for the clinician: Using the evidence* (3rd. ed., pp. 337–408). Burlington, MA: Jones and Bartlett.

Acknowledgments: The authors would like to thank the Board of Directors of Kemang Medical Care Mother and Child Hospital for the permission and support, and also to Arisma and Pica from Indonesia Breastfeeding Association for their help and support.

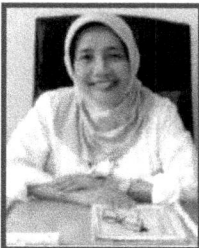

Asti Praborini, MD, Pediatrician, IBCLC, is a granny of a successful breastfeeding mother. Having 24 years of experience as a pediatrician convinced her that nothing is more important and valuable than breastfeeding for both mother and baby. As a national speaker, she continues to campaign for the benefit of breastfeeding despite the abundance of formula marketing. She built the first hospital-based lactation team in Indonesia that works ultimately to help mother breastfeed her baby. She is practicing frenotomy for anterior as well as posterior tongue-tie and lip-tie, established her method for hospitalization of nipple confusion, supplementation, adoptive nursing, and many others.

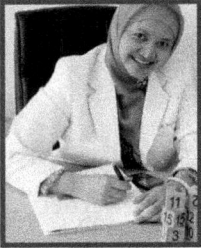

Hani Purnamasari, MD, Pediatrician, devoted her time in the lactation field after she found many babies had excessive weight loss and failure to thrive because of breastfeeding difficulties. She is joining the lactation team and now helping many mothers to achieve their breastfeeding goals. She is practicing frenotomy for anterior as well as posterior tongue-tie and lip-tie. Dr. Hani often speaks to promote the benefit of breast-feeding, and her best experience was sharing the same stage with Dr. Jack Newman (pediatrician) on Seminar and Workshop of Breastfeeding Update on Daily Practice, in Jakarta, Indonesia.

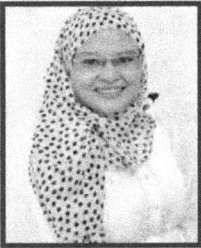

Agusnawati Munandar, MD, IBCLC, is a successful breastfeeding mother of two. She decided to enter the lactation field because she wants to embrace breast-feeding and help many mothers to succeed. She is working in a lactation clinic of baby-friendly hospitals and earned her International Board Certified Lactation Consultant degree in 2013. She is involved in a lactation team that helps many mothers to achieve their breastfeeding goals, such as practicing frenotomy for anterior as well as posterior tongue-tie and lip-tie, hospitalization for nipple confusion, supplementation, adoptive nursing, and others.

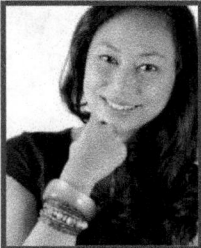

Ratih Ayu Wulandari, MD, IBCLC, entered the lactation field once she realized that breastfeeding mothers need help and support. Having experi-enced breastfeeding her tongue-tied baby helps her understand the pain and to support early frenotomy. She is now joining the lactation team and practicing frenotomy for anterior as well as posterior tongue-tie and lip-tie. She believes attachment parenting is the best way to nurture a child and shares her thoughts on her blog http://www.menjadiibu.com.

![USLCA logo]

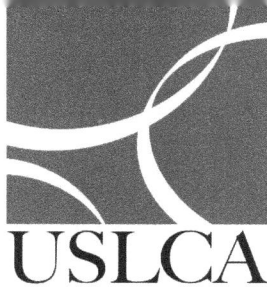

Acute, Subclinical, and Subacute Mastitis

Definitions, Etiology, and Clinical Management

Carmela Baeza, MD, IBCLC, RLC

Keywords: acute mastitis, subclinical mastitis, subacute mastitis, antibiotics, probiotics

There is a controversy about the origin, definition, and types of acute mastitis, breast pain, and their clinical management. This article reviews current definitions, bacteriological findings, their possible meanings, and their use in clinical settings as well as the latest evidence-based clinical management guidelines.

According to medical literature, mastitis is an inflammation of the breast that may or may not be accompanied with a bacterial infection (World Health Organization, 2000). The usual clinical definition of mastitis is a tender, hot, swollen, wedge-shaped area of breast associated with temperature of 38.5°C (101.3°F) or greater, chills, flulike aching, and systemic illness (Lawrence, 1990). This condition has also been classically referred to as acute or puerperal mastitis.

However, in clinical practice, we see inconsistencies in the concept and definition of mastitis. Recent discoveries about the composition of breast milk, its microbiological content, inflammatory and anti-inflammatory biochemical components, and the relationship of all these with the clinical findings have muddled the classical definition.

Kvist's (2010) review described this difference in criteria when defining mastitis in empirical studies about lactational mastitis. She reviewed 18 empirical studies published between 1998 and 2008. The conclusion was that there is no consensus or common criteria to define mastitis. In 10 of the reviewed articles, authors stated that mastitis could be either an inflammation or an infection. Four studies defined it as an infection, and another four did not clearly define it. Only 5 of the 18 studies included bacterial culture of the breast milk; the other 13 failed to state that milk culturing might be relevant. As for treatment options, antibiotics were strongly suggested in 4 articles, 4 stated that they may be needed in some cases, and the remaining 10 made no suggestion of the use of antibiotics for the management of mastitis.

These studies suggested several new possible etiologies of mastitis. Mastitis was described as a dysbiotic process, as the result of social, physiological, and pathological interactions. They identified it as a multifactorial syndrome.

Because of changing knowledge, diverse etiological theories, an abundance of varied clinical symptoms, and the range of people who diagnose mastitis (midwives, nurses, physicians, mothers, and lactation consultants), according to these studies, the concept of mastitis remains inconsistent.

Acute Lactational Mastitis

(Puerperal Mastitis)

The term acute in medical literature refers to "having a sudden onset, sharp rise, and short course" (Merriam-Webster Medical Dictionary, n.d.). The diagnosis of acute lactational mastitis is generally made clinically. It is characterized by localized, unilateral breast tenderness and erythema, accompanied by a fever of 101°F (38.5°C), malaise, fatigue, body aches, and headache in a breast-feeding mother (Lawrence & Lawrence, 2005; Wambach, 2003).

Management of Symptoms

The first step in the management of acute mastitis is frequent and efficient milk removal from the affected breast. This clear recommendation is well supported by evidence accumulated in the literature. In a randomized controlled trial (RCT) in Sweden (Kvist, Larsson, Hall-Lord, Steen, & Schalén, 2008), 85% of the 192 women in the breast-feeding group with acute mastitis symptoms responded favorably to effective draining of the breast and breast-feeding support and required no antibiotics. Milk was cultured from all the women in the study, the cases as well as the controls (consisting of 466 asymptomatic, healthy breastfeeding women). Interestingly, many women with potential pathogens, such as Staphylococcus aureus (S. aureus), coagulase-negative staphylococci (CNS), Group B streptococci (GBS), and Enterococcus faecalis (E. faecalis), were either in the asymptomatic group or recovered spontaneously. It is noteworthy that CNS were detected significantly more often in healthy controls, whereas S. aureus and GBS were significantly more frequent in the cases with acute mastitis symptoms.

Table 1. Clinical management of acute mastitis, based on the Academy of Breastfeeding Medicine 2014 Protocol

Initial 24 hours of fever	If 24 hours have passed and mother is not better, or has been growing worse	Milk culture should be considered if
• Frequent and efficient milk removal from affected breast • Rest, higher fluid intake • Symptomatic treatment of pain and fever (acetaminophen, ibuprofen . . .)	• Continue frequent and efficient milk removal from affected breast • Begin empirical antibiotic treatment for S. aureus • Symptomatic treatment of pain and fever (acetaminophen, ibuprofen . . .)	• There is no clinical response to antibiotic after 48 hours • Recurring mastitis • Hospital-acquired mastitis • Mother allergic to main antibiotics • Severe or "strange" mastitis

Osterman and Rahm (2000) studied 41 women who attended a breastfeeding service with symptoms of acute mastitis. Milk samples were taken upon arrival, and women were then managed with frequent and efficient milk removal and breastfeeding support. Only women whose symptoms did not resolve with this conservative approach were treated with antibiotics. When bacteriological culture results were received, women in the study were divided into two groups according to the results. For women in Group A, positive for CNS, mastitis resolved with frequent milk removal and rest. Women in Group B, positive mostly for S. aureus and also GBS, required antibiotics and suffered more complications, such as premature weaning, abscess, and fever. Thorough emptying of the breast alone, without need for antibiotics, was found to be curative for women with acute clinical mastitis and a positive milk culture for CNS.

The results of Kvist et al. (2008) and Osterman and Rahm (2000) indicate that management of acute mastitis should be based on the women's symptoms and not milk culture results. In addition, according to a recent Cochrane review, there is insufficient evidence from the RCTs currently available to evaluate the effectiveness of antibiotic therapy for lactational mastitis (Jahanfar, Ng, & Teng, 2013). Recommendation for first-line treatment with antibiotics should be considered carefully.

The most recent systematic review and evidence-based clinical management protocol was published by the Academy of Breastfeeding Medicine in the year 2014 (Amir & Academy of Breastfeeding Medicine Protocol Committee, 2014). The document reviews clinical management guidelines (Table 1), the evidence levels for treatment recommendations, main complications, and preventive measures.

This protocol confirms frequent and effective milk removal as the primary intervention in women with acute mastitis. Antibiotics should be started if symptoms are not improving within 12–24 hours or if the woman is acutely ill. The clinician should initially choose an antibiotic to cover S. aureus, the most frequent pathogen, as shown in Table

2 (Amir & Academy of Breastfeeding Medicine Protocol Committee, 2014; Jahanfar et al., 2013; Spencer, 2008)

Probiotics

Another management option that has been considered in the literature is the use of probiotics for acute mastitis treatment. There is only one study of a group of 20 women (Jiménez et al., 2008). These are women who had previous mastitis that did not respond well to antibiotic treatment. They had stopped taking antibiotics 2 weeks prior to the beginning of the study and presented with acute mastitis symptoms. They were assigned to two groups and given either probiotics or placebo. Midwives examined the mothers weekly. Although the results were promising (local inflammation and flulike signs disappeared in the probiotic group, clinical signs persisted in the placebo group), the study does not specify if the mothers did or did not receive other interventions such as counseling, aid with positioning and latch, frequent milk removal, or topic treatment for their nipple wounds. This study, because of its small size, the clinical characteristics of the mothers and other criteria is insufficient to demonstrate that probiotics can be used as an effective alternative to antibiotics for the treatment of acute mastitis.

Subclinical Mastitis

The term subclinical in medical literature refers to "not detectable or producing effects that are not detectable by the usual clinical signs" (Merriam-Webster Medical

Dictionary, n.d.). Subclinical mastitis (SCM) is an inflammatory condition of the lactating breast that is thought to be caused by poor lactation practice, milk stasis, and infections. SCM is typically diagnosed as either elevated breast milk sodium (16 mmol/L) or sodium/potassium ratio (Na/K ratio . 1.0; Morton, 1994). It is, by definition, asymptomatic and therefore cannot be detected by any clinical signs in the mother.

Table 2. Antibiotic Treatment Recommendations for Acute Mastitis		
Recommended Antibiotic	Dose	Duration of Treatment
Dicloxacillin or	500 mg PO QID	10–14 days
Cephalexin or	500 mg PO QID	10–14 days
Amoxicillin clavulanate	500 mg PO TID or 875 mg PO BID	10–14 days
If beta-lactam allergy:		
Clarithromycin	500 mg PO BID	10–14 days
If suspected methicillin-resistant *Staphylococcus aureus* (MRSA) infection:		
Clindamycin or	300 mg PO TID	10–14 days
Trimethoprim sulfamethoxazole	1 DS tablet PO BID	10–14 days

Note: PO = per orem; QID = four times a day; TID = three times a day; BID = two times a day; DS = double strength.

In the dairy industry, cows diagnosed with SCM produce less milk and therefore the diagnosis of SCM is of utmost importance. In human lactation, however, little is known about the effects of SCM on breast milk composition. The main interest of SCM in humans is the observation that among women infected with HIV, SCM is associated with increased milk HIV viral load (Kasonka et al., 2006; Willumsen et al., 2003). In some studies, SCM is associated with poor infant weight gain in lower stratus populations (Filteau et al., 1999; Kasonka et al., 2006). However, Flores and Filteau (2002) concluded that in their group of Bangladeshi women, a simple lactation counseling intervention could improve lactation practice and, as a consequence, SCM. In a more recent article, Aryeetey, Marquis, Brakohiapa, Timms, and Lartey (2009) were unable to demonstrate a difference in breast milk intake among infants whose mothers had SCM compared to those whose mothers did not. More studies are needed to confirm if correct breastfeeding support is the optimal management tool for these mother–baby pairs.

Subacute Mastitis

The term subacute in medical literature refers to "falling between acute and chronic in character especially when closer to acute" (Merriam-Webster Medical Dictionary, n.d.). The term subacute mastitis (SAM) is widely used in the dairy industry and animal research. Recently, the concept of subacute mastitis has appeared in texts pertaining to human lactation, introduced by Rodriguez and his group from the Nutrition, Bromatology, and Food Technology Department of the Veterinary Faculty at Complutense University in Madrid (Arroyo et al., 2010; Carrera et al., 2012; Jiménez et al., 2015). However, the authors themselves do not give a clear, single definition for subacute mastitis. In their 2010 study, they describe subacute mastitis as "inflammation of the breast and painful breastfeeding" (Arroyo et al., 2010). In a later article, they described it as "local pain, more or less intense, that feels like needles, cramps or burning, without visible redness (or very slight) and with no general symptoms" (Carrera et al., 2012). Finally, in their 2015 study, they define subacute mastitis as "burning/needle-like pain and engorgement" (Jiménez et al., 2015).

In classic human lactation literature, similar clinical descriptions have been used when referring to chronic mastitis, chronic/deep breast pain, and ductal thrush/candidiasis. Therefore, it does not seem that the term subacute mastitis helps to clear the current panorama.

Conclusion

The definition of mastitis remains inconsistent. New terms such as subclinical and subacute mastitis have yet to prove their usefulness. The etiology of mastitis may be inflammatory, infectious, multifactorial, or based on a bacterial imbalance that we cannot clearly interpret. However, despite these barriers, the clinical management of acute mastitis is well-defined and supported by evidence: frequent and efficient milk removal from the affected breast, breastfeeding support, and adequate antibiotic therapy only in cases that do not resolve with conservative measures.

References

Acute. (n.d.). In *Merriam-Webster medical dictionary*. Retrieved from http://www.merriam-webster.com/medical/acute

Amir, L., & Academy of Breastfeeding Medicine Protocol Committee. (2014). ABM clinical protocol #4: Mastitis, revised March 2014. *Breastfeeding Medicine, 9*(5), 239–243. http://dx.doi.org/10.1089/bfm.2014.9984

Arroyo, R., Martín, V., Maldonado, A., Jiménez E., Fernández L., & Rodríguez J. M. (2010). Treatment of infectious mastitis during lactation: Antibiotics versus oral administration of Lactobacilli isolated from breast milk. *Clinical Infectious Diseases, 50*(12), 1551–1558.

Aryeetey, R., Marquis, G. S., Brakohiapa, L., Timms, L., & Lartey, A. (2009). Subclinical mastitis may not reduce breastmilk intake during established lactation. *Breastfeeding Medicine, 4*(3), 161–166. http://dx.doi.org/10.1089/bfm.2008.0131

Carrera, M., Arroyo, R., Mediano, P., Fernández, L., Marín, M., & Rodriguez, J. M. (2012). Lactancia materna y mastitis. Tratamiento empírico basado en la sintomatología y los agentes etiológicos [Breastfeeding and mastitis: Empirical treatment based on symptoms and etiological agents]. *Acta Pediátrica Español, 70*(6), 255–261.

Filteau, S. M., Rice, A. L., Ball, J. J., Chakraborty, J., Stoltzfus, R., de Francisco, A., & Willumsen, J. F. (1999). Breast milk immune factors in Bangladeshi women supplemented postpartum with retinol or beta-carotene. *American Journal of Clinical Nutrition, 69*, 953–958.

Flores, M., & Filteau, S. (2002). Effect of lactation counselling on subclinical mastitis among Bangladeshi women. *Annals of Tropical Paediatrics, 22*(1), 85–88.

Jahanfar, S., Ng, C. J., & Teng, C. L. (2013). Antibiotics for mastitis in breastfeeding women. *Cochrane Database of Systematic Reviews*, (2), CD005458. http://dx.doi.org/10.1002/14651858.CD005458.pub3

Jiménez, E., de Andrés, J., Manrique, M., Pareja-Tobes, P., Tobes, R., Martínez-Blanch, J. F., . . . Rodríguez, J. M. (2015). Metagenomic analysis of milk of healthy and mastitis-suffering women. *Journal of Human Lactation, 31*(3), 406–415. http://dx.doi.org/10.1177/0890334415585078

Jiménez, E., Fernández, L., Maldonado, A., Martín, R., Olivares, M., Xaus, J., & Rodríguez J. M.. (2008). Oral administration of Lactobacillus strains isolated from breast milk as an alternative for the treatment of infectious mastitis during lactation. *Applied and Environmental Microbiology, 74*(15), 4650–4655. http://dx.doi.org/10.1128/AEM.02599-07

Kasonka, L., Makasa, M., Marshall, T., Chisenga, M., Sinkala, M., Chintu, C., . . . Filteau, S. (2006). Risk factors for subclinical mastitis among HIV-infected and uninfected women in Lusaka, Zambia. *Paediatric and Perinatal Epidemiology, 20*, 379–391.

Kvist, L. J. (2010). Toward a clarification of the concept of mastitis as used in empirical studies of breast inflammation during lactation. *Journal of Human Lactation, 26*(1), 53–59. http://dx.doi.org/10.1177/0890334409349806

Kvist, L. J., Larsson, B. W., Hall-Lord, M. L., Steen, A., & Schalén, C. (2008). The role of bacteria in lactational mastitis and some considerations of the use of antibiotic treatment. *International Breastfeeding Journal, 3*, 6. http://dx.doi.org/10.1186/1746-4358-3-6

Lawrence, R. A. (1990). The puerperium, breastfeeding, and breast milk. *Current Opinion in Obstetrics & Gynecology, 2*, 23–30.

Lawrence, R. A., & Lawrence, R. M. (2005). Management of the mother-infant nursing couple. *In Breastfeeding: A Guide for the Medical Profession (6th ed., pp. 255–316)*. St. Louis, MO: Mosby.

Morton, J. A. (1994). The clinical usefulness of breast milk sodium in the assessment of lactogenesis. *Pediatrics, 93*, 802–806.

Osterman, K. L., & Rahm, V. A. (2000). Lactation mastitis: Bacterial cultivation of breast milk, symptoms, treatment, and outcome. *Journal of Human Lactation, 16*(4), 297–302.

Spencer, J. P. (2008). Management of mastitis in breastfeeding women. *American Family Physician, 78*(6), 727–731.

Subacute. (n.d.). *In Merriam-Webster medical dictionary.* Retrieved from http://www.merriam-webster.com/medical/subacute

Subclinical. (n.d.). *In Merriam-Webster medical dictionary.* Retrieved from http://www.merriam-webster.com/medical/subclinical

Wambach, K. A. (2003). Lactation mastitis: A descriptive study of the experience. *Journal of Human Lactation, 19*(1), 24–34.

Willumsen, J. F., Filteau, S. M., Coutsoudis, A., Newell, M. L., Rollins, N. C., Coovadia, H. M., & Tomkins, A. M. (2003). Breastmilk RNA viral load in HIV-infected South African women: Effects of subclinical mastitis and infant feeding. *AIDS, 17*, 407–414.

World Health Organization. (2000). *Mastitis: Causes and management.* Geneva, Switzerland: Author.

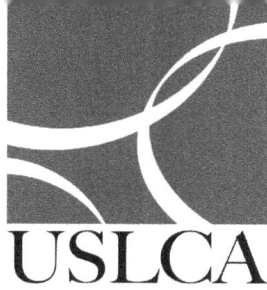

Chronic Mastitis, Mastalgia, and Breast Pain

A Narrative Review of Definitions, Bacteriological Findings, and Clinical Management

Carmela Baeza, MD, IBCLC, RLC

Keywords: mastitis, chronic breast pain, lactational mastalgia, antibiotics, probiotics

Whereas the management of acute mastitis seems clear, there is little scientific evidence to support management of chronic mastitis/breast pain. This article reviews bacteriological findings, their possible meanings, and their use in clinical settings. Clinical experience, newer and more accurate microbiological techniques, and the growing knowledge about our metagenome have many insights to offer.

Chronic mastitis is also known as chronic breast pain, deep breast pain, or chronic breast inflammation. However, there is no clear definition of any of these terms. Generally, in lactation literature, chronic mastitis refers to a lasting breast pain with no evidence of acute inflammation, such as erythema, warmth, or induration. The pain is described in various ways, often as deep, shooting pain, or burning sensation in one or both breasts that may happen during or between feeds. It may, or may not, be associated with nipple pain or nipple wounds (Betzold, 2007; Eglash, Plane, & Mundt, 2006; Witt, Mason, Burgess, Flocke, & Zyzanski, 2014). For simplicity, in this article, we will refer to this group of symptoms as lactational mastalgia (the suffix—itis in mastitis implies inflammation or infection; mastalgia is the medical term for breast pain). The broad spectrum of symptoms makes it likely that lactational mastalgia is not one single entity but a group of diverse conditions with diverse etiologies and with varying clinical manifestations.

Mastalgia is also found in nonlactating women, the pain described as "drawing," "burning," "achy," and "sore" (Smith, Pruthi, & Fitzpatrick, 2004). Therefore, the cause of mastalgia cannot be always ascribed to breastfeeding difficulties, which makes the etiology of the pain even more difficult to establish.

Management of Lactational Mastalgia

The most frequent cause of lactational mastalgia in breast-feeding women seems to be milk stasis or inadequate draining of the breast (Betzold, 2007; World Health Organization [WHO], 2000).This may be because of latch difficulties of diverse origins such as anatomical problems of mother's nipple and/or breast and anatomical or functional difficulties in the baby's latch/sucking ability.

Other factors resulting in poor draining include rapid weaning, oversupply, blocked ducts, missed feedings, external mechanical pressure on the breast, or incorrect hand/pump draining technique. Mastalgia may relate to the relative diameter of the milk ducts: the wider the ducts, the more severe the pain, as has been seen in ultrasound studies (Walker, 2010).

Several studies and clinical observations make us suspect other etiologies of lactational mastalgia, which may be a cause on their own or may be contributing to the milk stasis. These may include referred pain caused by nipple trauma secondary to an inadequate latch (Amir et al., 2013; Ellis, 1993; Hopkinson, 1992), musculoskeletal (pectoral/cervical thoracic muscle contraction secondary to strain, fear of painful latch, or unergonomic breastfeeding positions; Kernerman & Park, 2014; Thorley, 2005), or emotional in origin as also occurring in nonbreastfeeding women (Colegrave, Holcombe, & Salmon, 2001).

This pain requires thorough evaluation, a close observation and follow-up, and emotional support by a board-certified lactation consultant. Regardless of the presumed etiology, the basic treatment is consistent: effective milk drainage, breastfeeding support, and comfort measures for the mother (Betzold, 2007). While maintaining these three key interventions, the clinician can then address the etiological issues suspected (Table 1). A detailed history, evaluation of both mother and baby, and observation of a feed are necessary to unravel the cause/ causes of lactational mastalgia in each dyad.

Breast Pain, Candida and Bacteria: The Microbiological Debate

For many years, the main hypothesis was that lactational mastalgia is caused by Candida albicans, although recent studies on this issue show conflicting results. In a systematic review of seven studies of women with deep breast pain, Betzold (2012) concluded that evidence points to an infectious origin, either by C. albicans or Staphylococcus aureus.

Table 1. Management of Lactational Mastalgia*

Management of Lactational Mastalgia		
Basic management: Maintain while working on the etiological issues.		
1. Frequent, regular, and efficient drainage of the breast (baby, hand, or pump)		
Aim for 8–12 adequate feeds/expressions per 24 hours. Permit 3–4-hour stretch of sleep once per 24 hours.		
2. Support and encouragement		
3. Comfort measures (warmth, massage, analgesia)		
Suspected Etiology	**Action to Take as IBCLC**	**Referral**
Inadequate draining of breast	Correct latch/position. Correct infant anatomical/functional difficulties. Correct milk expression technique.	Refer to MD, CST, OT or other specialist you consider the infant to need
Referred pain from nipple trauma	Correct cause of nipple trauma.	
Muscular/skeletal problems	Correct unergonomic breastfeeding positions.	If not enough, Refer mother to physical therapist
Thoracic constriction-like symptoms	Pectoral muscle stretches	If not enough, Refer mother to physical therapist
Infectious origin	Milk culture	If positive, refer to MD for antibiotic/antifungal treatment.
Vasospasm	Comfort measures, correct latch.	If not enough, refer to MD for nifedipine.
Emotional issues	Support, counseling, Omega 3, sunlight, exercise	If not enough, refer to mental health specialist.
Mastodynia (hormonal related mastalgia)	Inform woman. Support	
Multifactorial	Take all actions needed. Can try alternative ideas (acupuncture, probiotics, homeopathy, etc.)	
You are unsure		Refer to another IBCLC.
Medical issues (costochondritis, necrotizing fasciitis, breast cancer, etc.)		Refer to MD with your suspicions.

Note. MD = medical doctor; CST = craneosacral therapist; OT = occupational therapist.

*Betzold, 2007; Kendall-Tackett, 2007; Kernerman & Park, 2014; Strong & Mele, 2013; Thorley, 2005.

A few small studies have demonstrated that the milk cultures among women with lactational mastalgia are more likely to reveal bacterial pathogens than candidiasis (Amir et al., 2013; Eglash et al., 2006). The latest studies, which use more modern techniques, find no trace of C. albicans in human milk (Hale, Bateman, Finkelman, & Berens, 2009; Jiménez et al., 2015). Clearly, further research is required to ascertain if C. albicans can be responsible for some cases of lactational mastalgia.

Delgado et al. (2009) propose that disruption in the normal bacterial flora balance in breast milk could lead to coagulase-negative staphylococci (CNS; mainly Staphylococcus epidermidis) overgrowth, and this overgrowth would be the cause of lactational mastalgia. This theory, however, has not been confirmed by other studies.

In a prospective, descriptive case control study, Witt, Mason, et al. (2014) detected a significant elevation of S. aureus in the subjects group (breastfeeding mothers with chronic mastalgia) as compared to the control group (asymptomatic breastfeeding mothers). Both the cases and the controls had similar levels of CNS. The authors point out that, in the case group, the higher the count of S. aureus in a mother, the lower her CNS and vice versa. "This inverse relationship between S. aureus and CNS growth," the authors conclude, "does not support a pathogenic role for coagulase-negative staphylococci." The results do support, however, a pathogenic role of S. aureus in chronic mastalgia, as other studies have (Eglash et al., 2006; Kvist, Larsson, Hall-Lord, Steen, & Schalén, 2008). Therefore, the current hypothesis is that S. epidermidis may be normal, health-promoting flora in the mammary microbiota. In his 2003 paper, Heikkilä and Saris (2003) observed that commensal milk bacteria (mainly S. epidermidis, Streptococcus salivarius, and Streptococcus mitis according to his study) have the capacity to suppress or diminish S. aureus growth. He also affirms that lactobacilli have an antimicrobial role, although only 10% of milk isolates had these bacteria. Therefore, CNS are the most abundant antimicrobials in breast milk.

More recently, Altuntas (2015) isolated, characterized, and evaluated the antimicrobial effect of S. epidermidis strains from different human milk samples. He observed that S. epidermidis has much activity against E. coli and Listeria monocytogenes. He also observed that all strains of S. epidermidis are active against S. aureus. Finally, he observed that, although probiotic microorganisms have antimicrobial activity, they were scarce in the human milk samples he studied.

Therefore, according to current available information, the most frequent cause of infectious lactational mastalgia seems to be S. aureus. There is doubt about C. albicans being a cause of lactational mastalgia, and it seems that CNS may play a protecting role and not a pathological one.

Based on these findings, several questions arise for the clinician. Should the milk of women with lactational mastalgia be cultured? If so, when? How should the results be interpreted? And what treatment should be implemented?

When to Culture Milk Samples

There are no current evidence-based guidelines to answer this question. The information available from cited authors (Betzold, 2012; Eglash et al., 2006; Witt, Burgess, Hawn, & Zyzanski, 2014; Witt, Mason, et al., 2014) suggests that cultures should be taken from women with lactational mastalgia who do not respond to conservative treatment (good lactation management and support, comfort measures).

How to Interpret Culture Results

We also have no evidence-based guidelines as to how to interpret milk culture results from women with lactational mastalgia. Existing guidelines are used by milk banks to screen for contamination of donated milk. An option for clinicians assisting mothers with lactational mastalgia is to use one of these guidelines as a baseline in interpreting culture results. For example, the National Institute for Health and Care Excellence clinical guideline CG93 Donor milk banks: Service operation revised in 2014 (National Institute for Health and Care Excellence, 2010) states that pooled donated milk is considered contaminated if the colony forming unit (CFU) counts are above 100,000 CFU/ml of total microorganisms, 10,000 CFU/ml of Enterobacteriaceae, or 10,000 CFU/ml of S. aureus. In Witt, Burgess, et al.'s (2014) study, all cases with S. aureus and pain had more than 10,000 CFU/ml. However, one mother in the control group had a higher count of S. aureus and was asymptomatic. Other studies confirm that many healthy breastfeeding women have potentially pathogenic bacteria in their breast milk and remain asymptomatic (Hunt et al., 2011; Kvist et al., 2008).

How to Treat When Infectious Lactational Mastalgia is Suspected

It seems logical, while we await for further evidence on this issue, to act on microbiological results according to women's clinical symptoms and evolution, with a close follow-up to help detect those in need of antibiotics. In these cases, oral antibiotics matched to breast milk culture may significantly decrease pain and is not associated with increased complications (Kvist et al., 2008; Witt, Burgess, et al., 2014).

Probiotics for Lactational Mastalgia

The global market for probiotics has risen vertiginously over the last decade (Transparency Market Research, 2015). In some European countries, the market for probiotics for breastfeeding women is now on the rise.

The proposed use for these products is treatment of breast pain and prevention of mastitis, as can be seen in product web pages (see product web page in reference list). However, when reviewing the use of probiotics for the treatment of lactational mastalgia, we find no clear evidence in the only published study (Arroyo et al., 2010). In this article, 352 women with "breast inflammation and pain during breastfeeding" (termed subacute/subclinical mastitis by the authors) were studied. The women were divided into three groups: two for probiotic and one for antibiotic. At the end of the 21-da intervention, the women in the probiotic groups had less pain. However, the study is not blind and the clinical design of the study is unclear. There is no control in the study for other factors that might have affected the results, such as breastfeeding support received by the mothers during those 21 days. Also, some of the mothers in the antibiotic group were not receiving adequate antibiotics for S. aureus. Finally, the authors disclose that some of the funds for this study came from noncode compliant industries as part of the FUN C FOOD group (Consolider Fun C Food, 2010), so it is not clearly an independent study.

At this time, there is not enough evidence to support the use of probiotics in the management of mastitis or breast pain. More studies are required. As we have discussed, levels of lactobacilli do not seem to be naturally high in breast milk. In a very recent study, a Spanish group confirmed, with a very sensitive technique, a low presence of lactobacilli and bifidobacteria in a group of 20 women (Jiménez et al., 2015). The implications of artificially rising these levels by giving oral probiotics have to be carefully considered.

Conclusion: The Need to Learn More

Our main difficulty arises from our lack of knowledge about normal human milk microbiota. In a fascinating study, Hunt et al. (2011) characterized the diversity and temporal stability of bacterial communities in human milk. Her group used a newer technique (based on pyrosequencing of the 16S ribosomal RNA gene) than had previously been used. They studied milk samples collected at three time points over a 4-week interval from 16 asymptomatic breastfeeding women. They found a much greater diversity of bacteria than what had been previously reported.

They write that, as in other studies, the most frequent phylotypes are Streptococcus and Staphylococcus, and they also find Serratia and Propionibacterium. They state that "conversely, whereas previous work has identified Lactobacillus and Bifidobacteria as common, but minor members (2%–3% relative abundance) of milk microbiota, very few sequences from these phylotypes were observed in our samples" (p. 2). These conflicting findings may be because of genetic, cultural, or environmental differences in the women that were studied. If we take a look at Figure 1, where Hunt's main results are shown, we can observe the great diversity and intrapersonal and interpersonal variability of the 15 main bacterial genre of these 16 mothers. Similar results can be seen in the Jimenez et al. (2015) study, to an even greater extent because these authors do a metagenomic study and find not only bacterial DNA but also the genomes of archaea, virus, fungi, and protozoa. Hunt et al. (2011) reflect on the origin of the bacteria, because a great part of the Streptococcus and other genre such as Rothia are abundant in infant saliva. We know that when a child breastfeeds, there is a retrograde flow of saliva into the breast (Ramsay, Kent, Owens, & Hartmann, 2004). How does frequent milk removal change mother's microbiota? Why are some microbes pathogenic for some mothers but not for others? Does the child's microbiota regulate the mother's and in what way? What do the changes we observe in each mother's microbiota mean? Is the mother protecting the child or vice versa? Why do some mothers have a changing microbiota, whereas others have a stable one? Would we see the same variability or stability in their babies' saliva microbiota? Are we looking at a response to the environment or to changes in mother or baby's immunological state? These questions raise fascinating speculation.

Following these studies, Sam Ma and his group of bioinformaticists and medical ecologists (Sam Ma et al., 2014) used Hunt et al.'s (2011) information and studied, for the first time, the bacterial interactions within human milk using network analysis to visualize multivariate relationships. They describe two disconnected subnetworks, with diverse cooperation and inhibition relationships. It is a complex article but the conclusions are clear: the dynamic balance of human milk depends on the interaction of its different components, and of this system with the mother as a whole: her genetic, immunological, physiological, and demographic characteristics and the interaction with her infant's microbiome. We have much still to discover.

Citing Ward, Hosid, Ioshikhes, and Altosaar (2013, p. 10), "Perhaps, it is the diversity and/or sequences of DNA within the milk metagenome that is beneficial to infants, as opposed to any one specific bacterial genus or species."

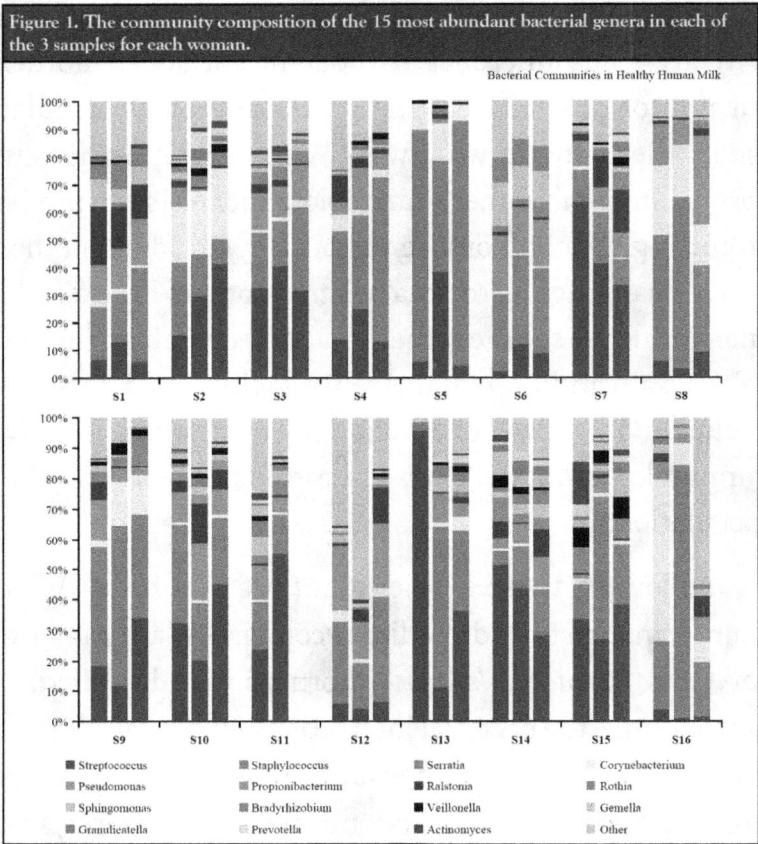

Figure 1. The community composition of the 15 most abundant bacterial genera in each of the 3 samples for each woman.

Image reproduced from "Characterization of the Diversity and Temporal Stability of Bacterial Communities in Human Milk," by K. M. Hunt, J. A. Foster, L. J. Forney, U. M. Schütte, D. L. Beck, Z. Abdo, . . . M. A. McGuire, 2011, PLoS One, 6(6), e21313. Copyright by Creative Commons Attribution License. Reprinted with permission.

The sciences that study human milk and human lactation are very young. We have before us an incredibly complex biological design that should be observed and studied to the best of our abilities. It has achieved the survival of our species for thousands of years. Manipulation of the human milk microbiota (by the excessive use of antibiotics or the indiscriminate use of probiotics) based on premature or non–evidence-based conclusions should be considered very carefully.

References

Altuntas, E. G. (2015). Isolation, identification and characterization of Staphylococcus epidermidis in human milk. *LWT Food Science and Technology, 60*, 36–41. http://dx.doi.org/10.1016/j.lwt.2014.07.012

Amir, L. H., Donath, S. M., Garland, S. M., Tabrizi, S., Bennett, C., Cullinane, M., & Payne, M. (2013). Does Candida and/or Staphylococcus play a role in nipple and breast pain in lactation? A cohort study in Melbourne, Australia. *BMJ Open, 3*, e002351. http://dx.doi.org/10.1136/bmjopen-2012-002351

Arroyo, R., Martín, V., Maldonado, A., Jiménez, E., Fernández, L., & Rodríguez, J. M. (2010). Treatment of infectious mastitis during lactation: Antibiotics versus oral administration of Lactobacilli isolated from breast milk. *Clinical Infectious Disease, 50*(12), 1551–1558.

Betzold, C. M. (2007). An update on the recognition and management of lactational breast inflammation. *Journal of Midwifery & Women's Health, 52*, 595–605.

Betzold, C. M. (2012). Results of microbial testing exploring the etiology of deep breast pain during lactation: A systematic review and meta-analysis of nonrandomized trials. *Journal of Midwifery & Women's Health, 57*(4), 353–364. http://dx.doi .org/10.1111/j.1542-2011.2011.00136.x

Colegrave, S., Holcombe, C., & Salmon, P. (2001). Psychological characteristics of women presenting with breast pain. *Journal of Psychosomatic Research, 50*(6), 303–307.

Consolider Fun C Food. (2010). *Alimentos funcionales* [Functional Foods]. Retrieved from http://www.alimentosfuncionales.org/empresa/empresas-integrantes/

Delgado, S., Arroyo, R., Jiménez, E., Marín, M., del Campo, R., Fernández, L., & Rodríguez, J. M. (2009). Staphylococcus epidermidis strains isolated from breast milk of women suffering infectious mastitis: Potential virulence traits and resistance to antibiotics. *BMC Microbiology, 9*, 82. http://dx.doi.org/10.1186/1471-2180-9-82

Eglash, A., Plane, M. B., & Mundt, M. (2006). History, physical and laboratory findings, and clinical outcomes of lactating women treated with antibiotics for chronic breast and/or nipple pain. *Journal of Human Lactation, 22*, 429–433.

Ellis, D. (1993). Post-feed breast pain: A case report. *Journal of Human Lactation, 9,* 182–183.

Hale, T. W., Bateman, T. L., Finkelman, M. A., & Berens, P. D. (2009). The absence of Candida albicans in milk samples of women with clinical symptoms of ductal candidiasis. *Breastfeeding Medicine, 4*(2), 57–61. http://dx.doi.org/10.1089/bfm.2008.0144

Heikkilä, M. P., & Saris, P. E. K. (2003). Inhibition of Staphylococcus aureus by the commensal bacteria of human milk. *Journal of Applied Microbiology, 95,* 471–478.

Hopkinson, J. (1992). Interfeeding breast pain: A case report. *Journal of Human Lactation, 8,* 149–151.

Hunt, K. M., Foster, J. A., Forney, L. J., Schütte, U. M., Beck, D. L., Abdo, Z., . . . McGuire, M. A. (2011). Characterization of the diversity and temporal stability of bacterial communities in human milk. *PLoS One, 6*(6), e21313.

Jiménez, E., de Andrés, J., Manrique, M., Pareja-Tobes, P., Tobes, R., Martínez-Blanch, J., . . . Rodríguez, J. M. (2015). Metagenomic analysis of milk of healthy and mastitis-suffering women. *Journal of Human Lactation, 31*(3), 406–415. http://dx.doi.org/10.1177/0890334415585078

Kendall-Tackett, K. (2007). A new paradigm for depression in new mothers: The central role of inflammation and how breastfeeding and anti-inflammatory treatments protect maternal mental health. *International Breastfeeding Journal, 2,* 6. http://dx.doi.org/10.1186/1746-4358-2-6

Kernerman, E., & Park, E. (2014). Severe breast pain resolved with pectoral muscle massage. *Journal of Human Lactation, 30*(3), 287–291.

Kvist, L. J., Larsson, B. W., Hall-Lord, M. L., Steen, A., & Schalén, C. (2008). The role of bacteria in lactational mastitis and some considerations of the use of antibiotic treatment. *International Breastfeeding Journal, 3,* 6. http://dx.doi.org/10.1186/1746-4358-3-6

National Institute for Health and Care Excellence. (2010). *Donor milk banks: Service operation.* Retrieved from https://www.nice.org.uk/guidance/CG93/chapter/Key-priorities-forimplementation

Ramsay, D. T., Kent, J. C., Owens, R. A., & Hartmann, P. E. (2004). Ultrasound imaging of milk ejection in the breast of lactating women. *Pediatrics, 113,* 361–367.

Sam Ma, Z., Guan, Q., Ye, C., Zhang, C., Foster, J. A., & Forney, L. J. (2014). Network analysis suggests a potentially 'evil' alliance of opportunistic pathogens inhibited by a cooperative network in human milk bacterial communities. *Sciemtific Reports, 5,* 8275.

Smith, R. L., Pruthi, S., & Fitzpatrick, L. A. (2004). Evaluation and management of breast pain. *Mayo Clinical Proceedings, 79,* 353–372.

Strong, G. D., & Mele, N. (2013). Raynaud's phenomenon, candidiasis, and nipple pain: Strategies for differential diagnosis and care. *Clinical Lactation, 4*(1), 21–27. http://dx.doi.org/10.1891/215805313806998499

Thorley, V. (2005). Latch and the fear response: Overcoming an obstacle to successful breastfeeding. *Breastfeeding Review, 13,* 9–11.

Transparency Market Research. (2015). Probiotic Market By Application (Food and Beverages, Dietary Supplements, Animal Feed) By End Users (Human Probiotics, Animal Probiotics)—Global industry analysis, size, share, growth and forecast 2014–2020. Retrieved from http://www.transparencymarketresearch.com/probiotics-market.html

Walker, M. (2010). *Breastfeeding management for the clinician: Using the evidence* (2nd ed.). Sudbury, MA: Jones & Bartlett Learning.

Ward, T., Hosid, S., Ioshikhes, I., & Altosaar, I. (2013). Human milk metagenome: A functional capacity analysis. *BMC Microbiology, 13,* 116. http://dx.doi.org/10.1186/1471-2180-13-116

Witt, A. M., Burgess, K., Hawn, T. R., & Zyzanski, S. (2014). Role of oral antibiotics in treatment of breastfeeding women with chronic breast pain who fail conservative therapy. *Breastfeeding Medicine, 9*(2), 63–72. http://dx.doi.org/10.1089/bfm.2013.0093

Witt, A., Mason, M. J., Burgess, K., Flocke, S., & Zyzanski, S. (2014). A case control study of bacterial species and colony count in milk of breastfeeding women with chronic pain. *Breastfeeding Medicine, 9*(1), 29–34. http://dx.doi.org/10.1089/ bfm.2013.0012

World Health Organization. (2000). *Mastitis: Causes and management.* Geneva, Switzerland: Author.

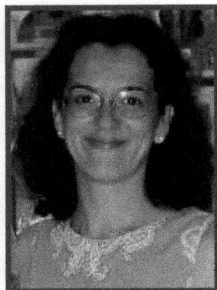

Carmela Baeza is a medical doctor specializing in family medicine. She became an IBCLC in 2005 and was a member of International Lactation Consultant Association a year before that. She has been a Baby-Friendly Hospital Initiative evaluator since 2006. She works in a private family health clinic, Raices, where she is in charge of the lactation program.

Over the past six years, she has coordinated 43 breastfeeding courses in which the educational team (four IBCLCs, including herself, two nurses, a pediatrician, and a midwife) has trained more than 3,000 doctors, midwives, and nurses from public hospitals in the Madrid area. They are a referent in breastfeeding training in Spain. Their page: http://www.centroraices.com/

She is part of a workgroup on ankyloglossia that is currently immersed in a clinical study to determine the effectiveness of frenotomy versus conservative treatment on posterior tongue-tie. She is also currently gathering data on the efficacy of oral Lactobacillus in women with chronic breast pain.

She coauthored (with Dr. Concha de Alba, IBCLC, MD) the chapter on breastfeeding in the book Pediatría Extrahospitalaria. Fundamentos Clínicos para Atención Primaria (Outpatient Pediatrics. Clinical Foundations for Primary Care), by M. T. Muñoz Calvo, M. I. Hidalgo Vicario, and J. Clemente Pollán, 2008, Madrid, Spain: Ergon.

She has published a book, Amar con los Brazos Abiertos, Ed Marova, 2013. It has two parts: The first is to make the science behind breastfeeding easy for parents to grasp, and the second is to address everyday parenting emotional issues that parents can turn from barriers into assets for their family growth. She has published breast-feeding articles in several popular mothering magazines in the last five years and has had several appearances in public national television on breastfeeding basics.

She organizes the yearly Hot Topics in Breast-feeding Conference at the prestigious College of Doctors in Madrid. Each year, we invite one single speaker to lecture us on the areas of her expertise for two consecutive days. Carmela does the live translation for the speakers.

Carmela is married and has five children.

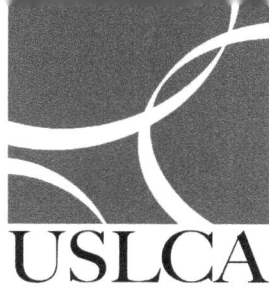

An Alternative Treatment

Using Ultrasound for Plugged Ducts—An Interview With Karen Lin

Barbara D. Robertson, MA, IBCLC, RLC

Keywords: plugged ducts, ultrasound, breastfeeding, mastitis

Mothers with persistent, reoccurring issues with plugged milk ducts in their breasts are usually in great amounts of pain and, therefore, at great risk for premature weaning. Why some mothers struggling with this issue seems unclear, but there is a treatment option that can offer immediate relief and perhaps a permanent resolution of these trouble areas in the breast. Using ultrasound treatment of the affected area of the breast is a highly effective, last resort treatment, but most IBCLCs do not have access to healthcare providers to refer to for this procedure. In this article, plugged duct treatments will be discussed with a focus on the specifics of using ultrasound for resolving this issue.

BR: Thank you for being willing to share this information. Karen, what brought you to see me in the first place?

KL: For returning to work . . . But I also was struggling with plugs. Every time my baby had a transition, I would get plugs. When she started solids, the plugs came back. When I went back to work, they came back . . . I had a little journal to keep track of my nursing so I would write "PDL" [plugged duct left] or "PDR" [plugged duct right] when I had them . . . It was a rough time.

BR: What made you think of using ultrasound on your plugs?

KL: I first found out about it through my breastfeeding doctor at the Breastfeeding Clinic through the University of Michigan . . . she said this is something you can try, but I don't know of any practitioners who do this. I called around, I called physical therapists because that is typically the person who uses ultrasound, and no one could help me, no one could give me direction . . . I actually went to our breast cancer center, they use diagnostic ultrasound, which is not the same thing as therapeutic ultrasound, but they didn't know anything about this. But in talking to one of my coworkers who is a physical therapist, she said you could just do this stuff on yourself. We have an ultrasound machine where I work, that's how I started experimenting with that.

BR: I know I talked to you about it as well, but I said I don't know who does it either . . . So, you heard this treatment possibility from multiple places and you had been thinking about it.

KL: Yes. Quite a few people had mentioned it, and this was the frustrating thing for me. A lot of people were telling me this is something you can try, but I couldn't find anyone who had any actual knowledge to guide me. Once I got some training, I pretty much just started doing it to myself when I went back to work. But 6 months later, my supervisor said, "We know that it is safe, it was not going to be harmful in any way. Go ahead and check out insurance codes." So, we have been offering this treatment for about 2 years, and there are so many people who are so thankful that it is an option, for those really stubborn plugs, or women like me who are just prone to them.

BR: Or you just keep getting a plug in the same place, over and over again. This treatment seems to be very helpful.

KL: Yes. There seems to be three different camps of women. The women who gets a plug, but rarely, just every once in a while. They know ultrasound treatment is appropriate, and I might see them once or twice over their whole breastfeeding career, so this could be over a year or two to treat an occasional stubborn plug. Then there's that type of women who, I believe it's the same plug that they are never able to fully eradicate with heat and of course, self-massage. But it's in the same exact spot. It's never resolved for more than an evening or day before it comes back, so I really think that's the same plug that's not resolved. And then there's the woman who is kind of classified like me, where they come every other week or every month, and it's in a different area each time. "Oh, it's the right breast now," "Oh, it's the left," "Oh it's under my nipple now," "Oh, it's near my armpit." And I say, "I feel so sorry for you!" These plugs can crop up anywhere. I feel like the latter two situations, the really stubborn plugs that they can't eradicate, or that poor woman who is really prone to them, where they just pop up anywhere, in any spot, I feel like using ultrasound is a really nice complement to what they are already doing.

BR: What did you personally do before you got into the ultrasound? What were the techniques were you using? What did you find to be effective and what didn't you not find to be effective?

KL: I did everything everyone told me to do, all the lactation consultants, all the word of mouth, online. I did self-massage. I did the back of an electric tooth brush. I did a hot shower. I did Epsom Salt baths. I did hot compresses. I did cold compresses to help with the swelling. I did dangle feeding. I feed my baby; you know what do they say? Point the chin towards where the plug is, and those two particular things, the dangle feeding and the pointing the chin. I have not met one person who has said that helped them.

BR: I agree. I haven't found it has helped much either.

KL: Everyone still tries it! So, lecithin was like the big savior. That really eased a lot of my issues. By the time a woman has gotten to my door, she has, most of them, have come through a lactation consultant, but for those weird situations where they haven't come to us that way, I'll say here's something you should know about. You should talk to your doctor about this. It's worth knowing about if you are getting recurrent plugs.

BR: What do you think about soy lecithin versus sunflower lecithin?

KL: I don't think I know enough about the difference.

BR: I have heard sunflower lecithin is better. Because I noticed in your handout you suggest lecithin, but that's not something that we suggest right away, but I guess by the time people come to you, it's like okay. You might want to give this a shot because they wouldn't be coming to you if they weren't struggling.

KL: Exactly. This program has really grown through lactation consultants. That's been the lovely thing. At a certain point, someone can say to these mothers, "You know these things [the easy things we try to resolve plugs], they aren't working for you! You've done what you are supposed to do, and perhaps we should take the next step." So, it's very rare that I get a woman with her first plug. And if I do, usually it's that woman who had a friend who had recurrent plugs. And the friend said, "Oh, this is what you should try," and she hasn't seen a lactation consultant. And that is incredibly rare. I prefer it the other way [Where the lactation consultant refers the mother to Karen]. I agree with you, most plugs are going to go away with normal therapies. This is for when those suggestions are not helping.

BR: Right. This is for moms that have chronic issues. Where did you find your information about how to go about doing this procedure?

KL: It's pretty much the power of the internet. I found a journal article (Lavigne & Gleberzon, 2012) [which had a protocol], but the protocol I follow is the one that they talk about on Jack Newman's site (Newman, n.d.). There's really not much of a difference between the two. The one suggests doing the ultrasound slightly longer, one is for 8 minutes and one is for 5, and slightly different megahertz, but not a substantial difference according to the physical therapist who taught me how to use the ultrasound machine. So that is where I found my information, and then my success using it on myself for my own issues really made me feel confident about helping others. OK, this is going to be helpful for other people.

BR: After you did this procedure to yourself, what was it like? Was it helpful right away? Did it take a while? Did you need multiple treatments? Tell me about that.

KL: You know you can have the bigger ones. I call those the stubborn ones. They're very tender right away, they get big right away. They hurt. Self-massage, you have to do it, but it's quite painful. Those, I have found with the ultrasound, I might have to do a second dose. Jack Newman's protocol says [do the ultrasound treatment] for 5 minutes for 1 day, and if it's not significantly better, do it for 5 minutes the next consecutive day, and the ultrasound, with the stubborn ones I call them, they would be resolve. Previously, these stubborn ones would linger for a week or so. It's shocking I never got mastitis! It would be the same situation. Same spot! I would think that I got on it, I'd work on it, but then I would go to sleep, and 4 hours later, I would wake up and there it is again. That kind of situation. But for the smaller ones where I could kind of feel it coming on, the area was getting tender, but it's not such a big lump, I would ultrasound it right away, and it wouldn't progress.

BR: How many treatments did you have to do to yourself? Because you said you were a chronic, multiple plug person, where they could crop up anywhere.

KL: By the time I was trained with using the ultrasound, I was already toward the path of weaning. My child was about 8 months old, so we were into solids, so I was well regulated. I would use it whenever I got a plug, but I wasn't having too many issues. But I would use it every time I got a plug.

BR: So how many times do you think you used it? Five times? Three times?

KL: Oh yeah. Like a handful. No more than that. The time it was particularly bad was when I went back to work. I was pumping and working 10 hours a day. My body freaked out!

BR: What does this procedure look like? Tell me in your own words. A mom comes in and what happens in your office?

KL: I will get a comprehensive picture of how frequently has [the mom] had to deal with this issue. When did this particular plug crop up? It's a little bit of a chatting at first. I want to make sure that I am understanding the situation. I also want to make sure that this mom has done all of the typical, conventional things first. I have never met someone who comes in and has not done at least five things [to try and resolve this issue], they say, this is what I do, and then I do this, I don't wear an underwire bra, and I don't do this. Just to make sure! So, we do that.

Then I specifically palpate the area and always ask about pain levels. I have to feel them. [I want to know] where are we at [painwise] when we start. Where are we at when we finish. And then we do the ultrasound. It's very easy; 5 minutes. A lot of times they say it feels like a little tingle, or they don't feel anything at all. What's easiest is if they take off their bra and top. I trained with an occupational therapist whose specialty is lymphedema, and together we developed some massage techniques that will also stimulate your lymphatic system, and the port that I focus on is the axilla, the armpit, which makes sense because it's the closest drain we can get to. [So after the ultrasonic treatment] we do light stroking, light massage, we're really trying to break that plug up, and afterward I will say, "Hey, if you can nurse now, if you can pump now, it's the time!"

BR: It sounds like most of the time it works. From what my clients have told me, it's like a miracle. If the mom does pump, does she ever see clumpy milk? Is this something

that moms might expect or have you not heard anything about this?

KL: I know with myself once after I cleared a plug once with my pump, and it was surprisingly, shockingly gross! It was like [the consistency of] whiteout!

BR: What have you now done to make this procedure available to other mothers?

KL: A lot of things! I think initially people either hadn't heard of this, see this was my frustration initially, I [work as a pediatric occupational] therapist, so I would be [working with] kids who have feeding difficulties, and not just at breast, they could be on the bottle. These kids would come, and these mothers are attempting to be exclusive pumpers, and quite a few would say to me, "Oh, I've had so many plugged ducts, lots of bouts of mastitis." And I'm thinking, we could have done something. Maybe it would have been successful. Maybe it wouldn't have. But it would have been something to try. Especially for those who wanted to try that path. But if you were trying to pump and you got a plugged duct, and that was your hold up, and you didn't know you could try ultrasound, that to me is sad.

KL: We had such a good response through our lactation consultation population, every one's on board. Our midwives through the U of M have all been on board. A problem is lactation consultants can't write referrals, and we need a referral. So, my biggest problem was getting a referral from the doctor in a timely manner to actually get these mothers in. Typically, it's an OB/GYN who's not familiar with this, they are hard to get a hold of, we have over 40 at the U of M. It's about education. I created this presentation, and I've been forcing myself to go to the clinics and present it, can I tell you about this. There are a lot of physical therapists who do pelvic floor work who didn't know about this. I am still working on getting the word out. That has been successful . . . Just through that, people are recognizing this is a really simple intervention to try with moms who are struggling with this problem. This is something anyone can offer. You just need that basic knowledge (see Table 1). So, there are bunch of different ambulatory clinics that are now ready to go. Aware, if a mom was to call and say, "I'm having this problem." So, if someone comes in, they can write that referral, and you can send them to us. You can have them walk right over to us. So, they are catching it quickly. The mothers are not having to suffer another day, or worse yet, take a hit to a milk supply that's maybe already suffering.

BR: Right. One of the major reasons women wean is pain. If you are suffering over and over again with these plugs, the odds of you weaning are high, and as you say, there is a treatment option. Are there any contraindications for a mother getting this treatment?

KL: Yes. The two major ones are if there is a suspicion that it may be anything other than a plugged duct. If there is concern for a tumor or a malignancy. I have a lot of patients come in and wonder if this is a possibility that this is what it could be. We typically tell them if there is a possibility, your doctor probably wouldn't write a referral for this [type of treatment]. They would be checking something else out. A plugged duct is pretty consistent as to what it looks like. The other contraindication is if there is an infection. I have had to tell mothers if it has developed into mastitis, "Are you on antibiotics?" They have to have been taking them for at least 48 hours, so the problem is resolving. "No more fever, you feel better, then we can ultrasound." [Another possible contraindication is for women who have had breast augmentation on the effected side.]

Table 1. Breast Self-Massage for Lactating Mothers

1. Use fingertips to softly stroke the clavicle (collarbone) from the neck outwards to the shoulders, keeping the bone between the middle and ring fingers. Repeat 5-10 times.

2. Using the same finger positioning and direction, apply circular pressure from the neck outwards to the shoulders. Repeat 5-10 times.

3. Place one hand behind the head and use the opposite hand's fingertips to apply 5-10 downward circular stokes to the breast, under the armpit.

4. On the same breast, cup one hand above and one hand below the breast. Use firm-gentle pressure to massage the breast in opposite directions for 5-10 counts.

5. Repeat #3 and #4 on the opposite breast.

6. Bend at the waist and dangle the head, arms, and breasts loosely towards the ground for a count of at least 5.

7. In this position, cup the breast with one hand above and one hand below the breast. Massage the breast by cupping one hand on top and one on the bottom of the breast for 5-10 counts.

8. Use one hand to apply 5-10 upward circular stokes to the breast, just under the armpit. Continue to make circular stokes around the base of the entire breast.

9. Repeat #7 and #8 on the opposite breast.

10. Return both arms to the "dangling" position, then slowly lift the torso and return to a standing position.

11. Roll shoulders backwards for a count of 10.

12. Lift both arms until hands meet above the head. Grasp the fingers of one hand with the other, then use this hand to pull the arm over, leaning at the waist.

13. Return to standing upright, then repeat #12 towards the opposite side.

14. Repeat #1.

BR: So, if a mother is worried, or perhaps the healthcare provider, that it is breast cancer, they would go to the breast cancer center first and get that assessed. And then if it is not cancer, yes, it is a plug, then they can come to you?

KL: Yes.

BR: Tell me about the procedure codes that you have created. You have this coded so it is covered by most insurance companies.

KL: Yes. Actually, it's an existing code. There were a bunch of codes out there. There's a code "Occlusion of the duct, comma, breast." There's another code, "Disorder of lactation." Those were preexisting ones that doctors were billing under for moms that were coming in with this issue. I plucked the ones that appeared to be most relevant. We are lucky enough to have an insurance checker, the referral coordinator, and she was good enough to call most of our major insurance providers and make sure these were considered a covered code. Those two cover what we work on and are thankfully, covered. Whenever I send out something to the doctor, I make sure to say, "Put down these codes; use one of these."

BR: Can you share with me what you send to doctors?

KL: Sure! I have a little sheet. [See handout.] The top part is occupational therapy, breastfeeding support, a little bulleted section for babies and one for mothers, and that's pretty much the plugged duct portion, and on the bottom of that I have the two diagnoses codes I suggest.

BR: Is there anything else you would like to share before we end?

KL: This has been a situation where you [as an IBCLC] know way more than me about all of this. I always feel like everyone else has given me so much information, I feel I'm just the person who put it in a package, all together.

BR: But you did. You actually did. You bothered to do it! So, you get credit for that!

KL: I feel you knew all this stuff, I just made in a place where people could actually come and access it. That's been the positive. You can take this and run with it.

BR: We can get this out to so many people. It's not like this is brain surgery, but people weren't putting it together and putting in practice so it will be nice to get this out.

KL: My hope is that one day, someone can come into their healthcare provider, and say, "This is what is going on, I have a chronic plug," and the provider will say, "Oh, it's not going away? This is what we can do."

BR: Thank you very much Karen for taking the time for sharing this with us!

References

Lavigne, V., & Gleberzon, B. J. (2012). Ultrasound as a treatment of mammary blocked duct among 25 postpartum lactating women: A retrospective case series. *Journal of Chiropractic Medicine, 11*(3), 170–178. Retrieved from http://www.ncbi.nlm.nih.gov/pmc/articles/PMC3437340/

Newman, J. (n.d.). Blocked ducts & mastitis. Retrieved from http://www.breastfeedinginc.ca/content.php?pagename=doc-BD-M

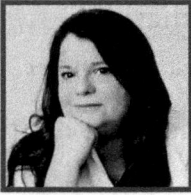

Barbara D. Robertson, IBCLC, has been involved in education for more than 28 years. She received a bachelor's degree in Elementary Education in 1988 and her master's in Education in 1995. Barbara left teaching elementary students in 1995 to raise her two children. Barbara is now the director of The Breastfeeding Center of Ann Arbor. Barbara has developed a 90-hour professional lactation training, a 20-hour course which fulfills the "Baby Friendly" education requirements, and is a speaker for hire on a wide variety of topics including motivational interviewing. Barbara volunteered for the United States Lactation Consultation Association (USLCA) as the director of Professional Development for 4.5 years. She is currently an associate editor for Clinical Lactation, a journal she helped create for USLCA. Barbara has free podcasts, a blog, and YouTube videos, which can all be found on her website http://bfcaa.com/. She has written many articles and created a phone app for working and breastfeeding mothers. She loves working with mothers and babies, helping them with breastfeeding problems in whatever way she can.

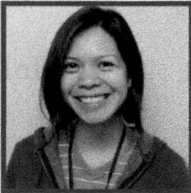

Karen Lin, OTRL, graduated with a Bachelor of Science degree in Occupational Therapy in 1999 and currently works in the University of Michigan Health System as a pediatric occupational therapist (OT). She expanded her area of service to include treatment of plugged milk ducts in 2013, after her own harrowing experience with plugged ducts.

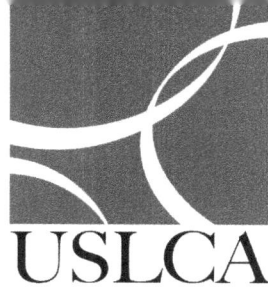

Management of Common Breastfeeding Problems

Nipple Pain and Infections: A Clinical Review

Tipu V. Khan, MD, FAAFP

Jennifer Ritchie, IBCLC, RLC

Keywords: breastfeeding; mastitis; human milk; exclusive breastfeeding; milk let-down

The U.S. Department of Health and Human Services Healthy People 2020 goal is to achieve a rate of breastfeeding at 12 months of age of 34.1%. Primary care providers are the first line in breastfeeding—from prenatal nipple evaluations to identifying and treating complications early. Breastfeeding conveys numerous benefits for both infant and mother. Currently, 77% of women attempt breastfeeding, but only 16% are still breastfeeding at 12 months of age. One of the top reasons for failure is lack of provider support when faced with breastfeeding problems. When the diagnosis is missed, complications can include hospitalization and cessation of breastfeeding. Understanding and being able to manage complications as well as having a team care approach involving an IBCLC and support group such as La Leche League are crucial in ensuring breastfeeding success.

Practice Recommendations/Strength of Recommendation (SOR)

A. Good-quality, patient-oriented evidence

B. Inconsistent or limited-quality, patient-oriented evidence

C. Consensus, usual practice, opinion, disease-oriented evidence, case series

» The U.S. Preventive Services Task Force (USPSTF) recommends interventions during pregnancy and after birth to promote and support breastfeeding (SOR B; Chung et al., 2008).

» Breastfeeding lowers rates of asthma, sudden infant death syndrome, types 1 and 2 diabetes, and obesity in infants (SOR A; Weng et al., 2013).

» Breastfeeding lowers rates of type 2 diabetes mellitus, PE1 breast and ovarian cancers, and postpartum depression in mothers (SOR A; Ip et al., 2007; Office on Women's Health, U.S. Department of Health and Human Services, & Womenshealth.gov, 2011).

» Minimal recommended time of breastfeeding is 6 months (SOR B; American Academy of Family Physicians [AAFP], 2012; American Academy of Pediatrics [AAP], 2013).

» Treat mastitis with antibiotics (SOR C; Crepinsek, Crowe, Michener, & Smart, 2010; Jahanfar, Ng, & Teng, 2013).

Benefits of breastfeeding to the child include strengthened immune system; easier digestion; and lower rates of asthma, obesity, sudden infant death syndrome, childhood cancers, and types 1 and 2 diabetes (Sor A, B, and C) (Weng et al., 2013). Benefits for the mother include less missed work; more physical contact and bonding; and lower rates of type 2 diabetes, breast cancer, ovarian cancer, and postpartum depression (Ip et al., 2007).

SOR A	SOR B	SOR C
• Breastfeeding lowers rates of asthma, sudden infant death syndrome, types 1 and 2 diabetes, and obesity in infants. • Breastfeeding lowers rates of type 2 diabetes mellitus, breast and ovarian cancers, and postpartum depression in mothers.	• The U.S. Preventive Services Task Force (USPSTF) recommends interventions during pregnancy and after birth to promote and support breastfeeding. • Minimal recommended time of breastfeeding is 6 months.	• Treat mastitis with antibiotics.

The American Academy of Family Physicians (AAFP) and the American Academy of Pediatrics (AAP) recommend 6 months of exclusive breastfeeding and a minimum of 12 months overall (AAFP, 2012; AAP, 2013). The World Health Organization (WHO) recommends exclusive breastfeeding for 6 months, but a longer 24-month period of supplemental breastfeeding because 24 months is the average time required for a child's immune system to mature (World Health Organization [WHO],). According to WHO, the global average from 2007 to 2014 for exclusive breast-feeding at 6 months is 36% (WHO,). The United States lags behind world averages for breastfeeding. According to the Breastfeeding Report Card, 16.4% of infants are exclusively breastfed at 6 months, and 27% are still breastfeeding at 12 months (Centers for Disease Control and Prevention, 2013).

Success at breastfeeding begins with education at preconception, each trimester, and postpartum (Chung et al., 2008). This includes evaluation of the breast and nipple as well as discussing breastfeeding at all prenatal visits. Educating the father of the baby prior to delivery can boost the initiation of breastfeeding by 33% (French, 2005). Choosing a breastfeeding-friendly hospital and access to trained lactation consultants, such as an IBCLC, are equally important (Rosen-Carole & Hartman, 2015).

Breast infections associated with lactation occur in 2%–10% of women and typically occur within the first 6 weeks postpartum (Committee on Health Care for Underserved Women, 2007). The infection manifests as painful swelling with overlying erythema. Women may experience fever, myalgias, and malaise. Infection begins as bacteria on the skin permeate through the nipple and infiltrate underlying stagnant milk, resulting in mastitis. Multiple factors increase the risk of lactational mastitis, including blockage of the milk duck and diminished drainage, oversupply of milk, infrequent feedings, nipple excoriation, maternal fatigue, and maternal malnutrition (Foxman, D'Arcy, Gillespie, Bobo, & Schwartz, 2002). Infection can be prevented as mothers employ proper breastfeeding techniques with frequent feeds and complete emptying of milk with each feed (Department of Child and Adolescent Health and Development, 2000). A proper latch technique, which can improve emptying of milk, is depicted in Figure 1. Notice the mother's C-grip on the breast and the infant's everted lips encompassing the majority of the areola, which results in a deeper latch.

The goal of this clinical review is to educate both primary care providers and clinicians to improve the outcomes of breastfeeding. By ultimately providing clinicians with the ability to assess and manage common postpartum breast complications, specifically breast infections, we hope to increase patient understanding, comfort, and likelihood of continued breastfeeding.

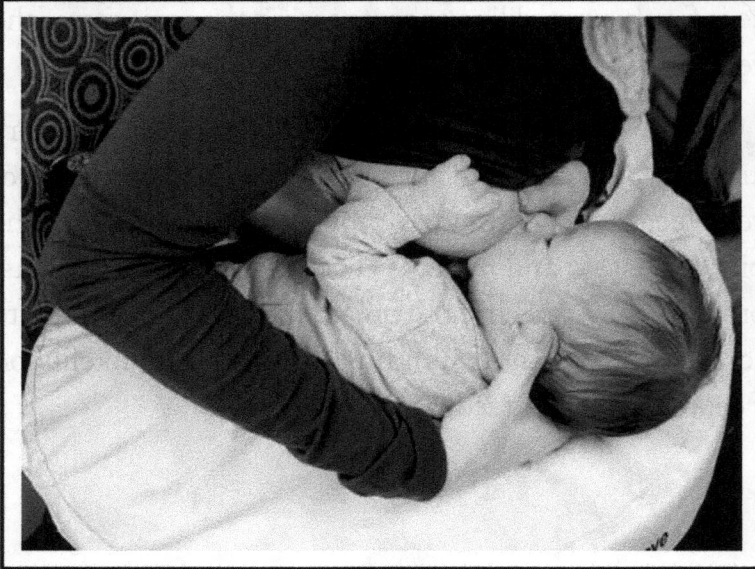

Figure 1. A proper latch involves wide flanged lips and deep penetration of the nipple-areolar complex into the soft palate. Maternal compression of the breast during latch as well as the use of a breastfeeding pillow may help in ensuring a deep and comfortable latch.

Nipple Pain

Although some nipple pain is common in the first few days of breastfeeding, sore nipples should not persist beyond this period and are often wrongly disregarded as a "normal" product of breastfeeding. Sore nipples may be because of abrasions that occur during feeding or from tight fitting clothing. These breaks in the skin predispose the mother to infections of the nipple as well as mastitis. To promote healing for noninfected cracked nipples, apply breast milk, air dry, and then apply nipple cream, such as lanolin between feedings (MorlandSchultz & Hill, 2005). Early intervention of skin breaks in the nipple is recommended to prevent secondary impetigo or candidiasis.

Assess for an improper latch or flat/inverted nipples as a common cause of nipple pain without infection. (Figure 2)

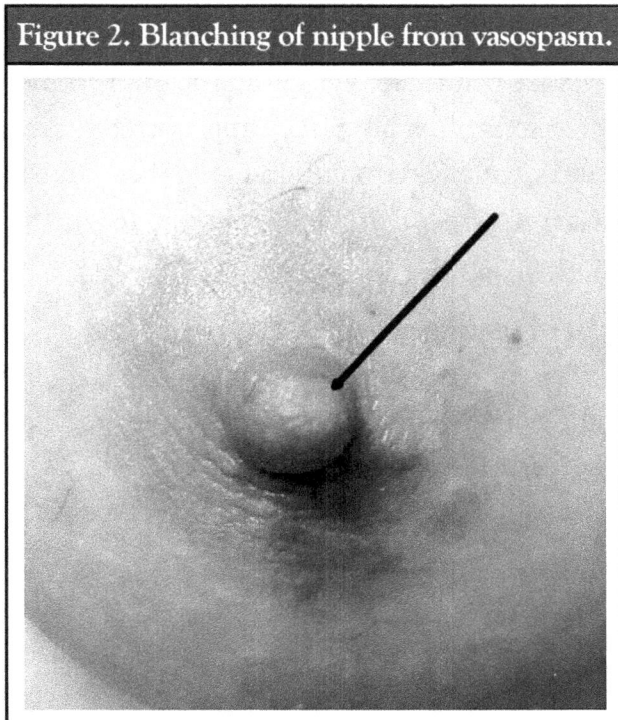

Figure 2. Blanching of nipple from vasospasm.

Consult with an experienced provider to evaluate latch depth with or without ultrasound and consider changing position during feeding. The use of a nipple shield may be helpful if indicated; however, it requires prompt follow-up to aid in weaning off the shield and limiting duration of use. A nipple shell is helpful to evert the nipple; however, this also requires prompt follow-up (Chakrabarti & Basu, 2011; La Leche League International, 2008). If pumping, have mother bring in her pump and flanges to ensure a proper fit. Evaluate the infant for ankyloglossia as a potential cause of nipple pain.

Often, vasospasm (Figure 2) can occur secondary to infection or intrinsic causes such as Raynaud's phenomenon, which presents as a burning sensation at the end of feeding. Heat packs are helpful for symptomatic improvement after feeds. Infections must be treated appropriately. In the case of Raynaud's, treat with nifedipine 5 mg thrice daily to limit spasm (Barrett, Heller, Stone, & Murase, 2013).

Occasionally, milk flow can become obstructed at the nipple pore creating a superficial milk blister (Figure 3). If the obstruction persists, this can lead to plugged ducts presenting as engorgement and painful lump. Encourage frequent feedings, warm compresses, and massage to improve removal of blockage (Lawrence et al., 2008).

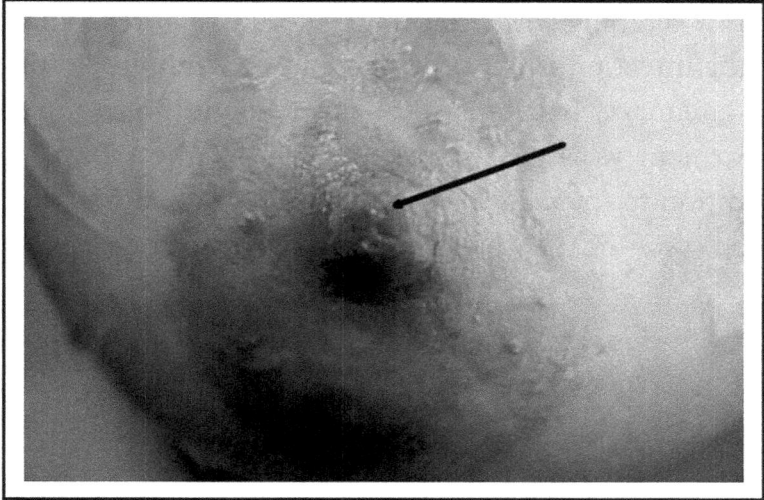

Figure 3. Plugged ducts. Note the blebs on the nipple.

Breast Infections

If an infectious cause is identified, thoroughly clean and sterilize all bottles, nipples, pacifiers, and pumping supplies by boiling them for 20 minutes daily. Wash all clothing in hot water to prevent reinfection. Keep areola clean and dry.

Impetigo

Most commonly from Staphylococcus aureus and group A beta-hemolytic streptococcus. Bacterial infections present as tender, cracked, honey crusted, and erythematous nipples (Figure 4). A nipple pore may also be blocked by colonization of Staphylococcus aureus infection and presents as a white pore (Figure 5; Livingstone, 1997). Begin

129

routine nipple hygiene with soap and water to remove any crusting. The patient can exfoliate with a washcloth after showers. The provider can try removing crusting by lightly scraping with an 18-gauge needle (Figures 6 and 7). If the infection is superficial, topical 2% mupirocin may be adequate. If extensive or not responding to topical treatment within 48 hours, begin systemic therapy in addition to topical treatment. See Table 1 for commonly used systemic therapies and their suggested dosages.

Figure 4. Impetigo of the nipple. Note the yellow crust and erythematous nipple from infection by *Staphylococcus aureus*.

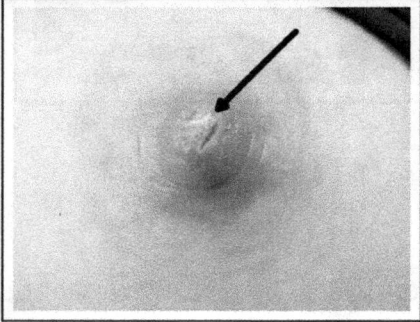

Figure 5. Pore colonization by *Staphylococcus aureus* presenting as a white papule with surrounding yellow crust.

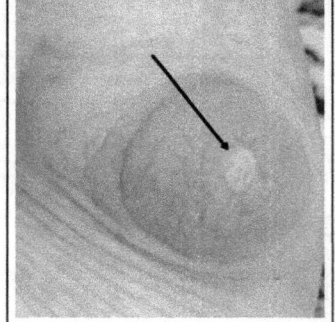

Figure 6. Severe impetigo before debridement now causing mastitis (surrounding erythema).

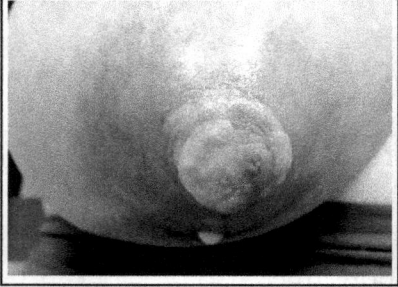

Figure 7. Same patient in Figure 6 post debridement treatment in clinic.

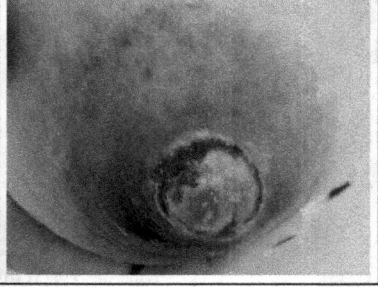

Candidiasis

It is often difficult to differentiate candidiasis versus impetigo of the nipple (Figure 8). Candidiasis may present as an exquisitely tender pruritic nipple but with minimal objective findings on exam other than superficial erythema. A dry dermatitis may be observed in some cases (Figure 9). A potassium hydroxide (KOH) scraping may assist in making the diagnosis if fungal remnants such as hyphae are seen on microscopy.

Table 1. Pharmacological Treatment of Impetigo		
Medication	Directions	Duration
Topical mupirocin 2%	Apply tid after feeds.	Until cleared
Oral dicloxacillin Oral cephalexin Oral erythromycin	500 mg every 6 hours	10 days

Note. tid = 3 times a day.

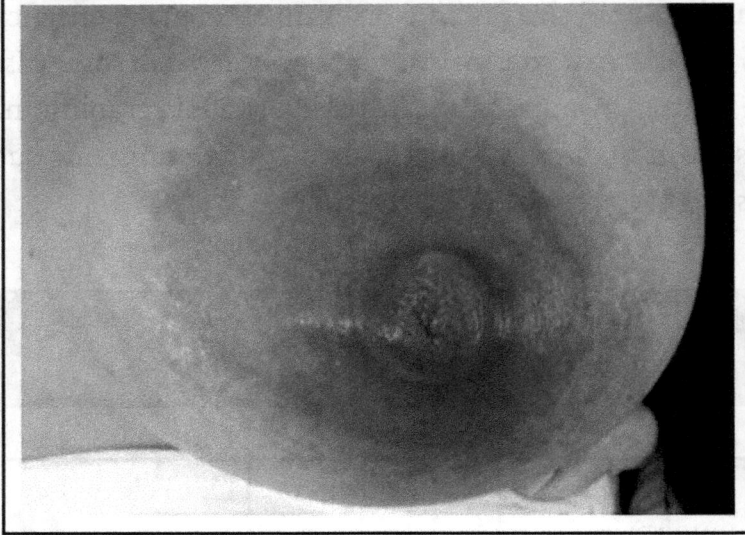

Figure 8. Candidiasis of the nipple. Tenderness, nipple pain, and erythema may be the only objective findings.

Once identified, the infant must also be treated to fully eradicate the infection with oral nystatin or fluconazole solution. Vice versa holds true—if an infant is diagnosed with oral candidiasis, the mother should be prophylactically treated even if no symptoms are present in the mother to prevent cross infection. Common treatment regimens for maternal candidiasis are listed in Table 2. Be sure to identify and treat other potential sources of candida such as vulvovaginal or infant diaper candidiasis.

Figure 9. Candidiasis of the nipple. Note the dry dermatitis and erythema.

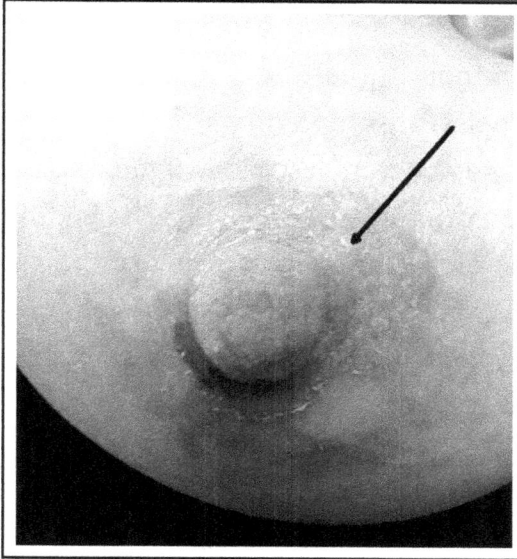

Table 2. Management of Maternal Candidiasis

Treatment	Dosing
Topical clotrimazole Topical miconazole Topical ketoconazole	Apply after each feed. Continue for 10–14 days after symptoms resolve.
Oral fluconazole	400 mg loading dose followed by 200 mg daily for 14–21 days
Vinegar solution	Mix 1 teaspoon of white vinegar in 1 cup of water. Apply after each nursing to nipple and allow to air dry.
Gentian violet (.25%–5% solution)	Apply to nipples twice daily for 3 days.

Note. For recurrent or refractory cases, oral therapy may be required.

Mastitis

Mastitis (inflammation of the breast) can be caused by numerous reasons, including infection or obstruction and is most common in the first 6 months of breastfeeding. Cracked nipples, missed feedings, oversupply of milk, tight fitting clothing, maternal stress/fatigue, and malnutrition are common causes (Academy of Breastfeeding Medicine, 2008). Most often, it affects one breast and presents as a red, tender lump or area of breast tissue along with fever, lumpy or stringy like milk, and malaise (Figures 10 and 11). In severe cases, purulent drainage may be evident.

A common cause of both mastitis and plugged ducts is inadequate emptying of the breast. Treatment requires routine emptying of the breast every 2 hours. Before nursing, apply warm compresses to help mobilize and dissolve clotted milk. Advise mothers to avoid tight fitting clothing. Consider cold compresses in-between feedings to help reduce pain and inflammation.

Prescribe appropriate analgesia as needed including nonsteroidal anti-inflammatory drugs (NSAIDs) to reduce inflammation. Have mother try different feeding positions to help fully empty the breast. Consider therapeutic ultrasound to provide deeper heat and initiate inflammatory tissue repair (Ritchie, 2013).

If mastitis is present more than 24 hours and conservative measures have failed, or the mother has a fever or is systemically ill, treat with antibiotics to cover Staphylococcus aureus, Streptococcus, Escherichia coli, and methicillin-resistant Staphylococcus aureus if appropriate for a 10–14 day course. Table 3 contains commonly used medications and their dosages for the treatment of infectious mastitis. Albeit there is a lack of evidence supporting or negating preventative strategies and treating mastitis, most clinicians opt to treat (Crepinsek et al., 2010; Jahanfar et al., 2013). In severe cases of mastitis or concern for systemic inflammatory response syndrome or Sepsis, admit for inpatient management and consider surgical consult for incision and drainage. Remember to consider inflammatory breast cancer as a cause. Perform breast milk culture for refractory or recurrent cases. Continue to nurse unless an abscess is drained.

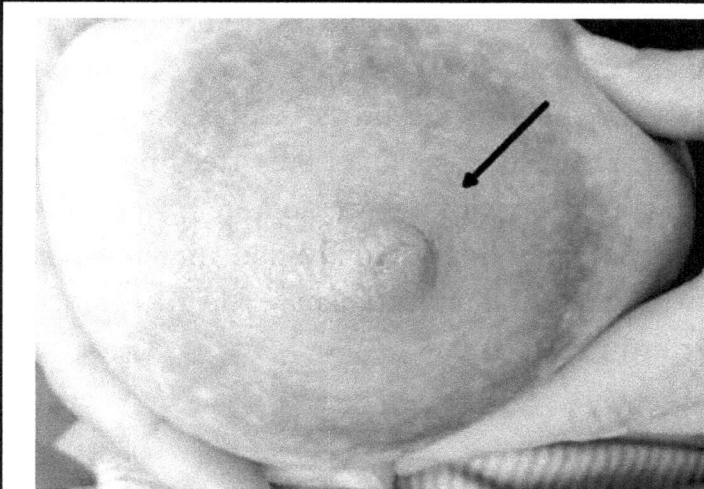

Figure 10. Developing mastitis from an untreated bacterial nipple infection.

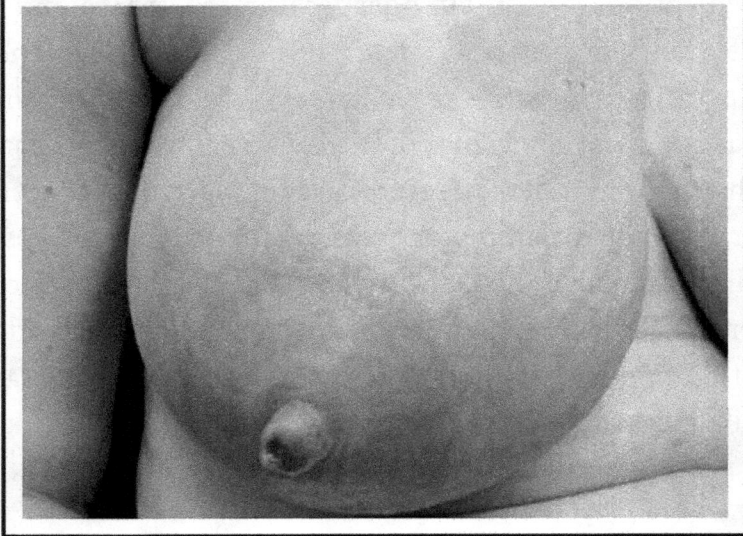

Figure 11. Moderate infectious mastitis.

Conclusion

Common breastfeeding problems are often underdiagnosed and untreated by clinical providers. Without proper support, mothers facing breastfeeding complications will often resort to cessation of breastfeeding. This may also be associated with missed time from work, anxiety, frustration, and depression. Ensuring appropriate follow-up and early intervention may help further increase breastfeeding success.

Table 3. Treatment of Infectious Mastitis		
Treatment	Dosing	Notes
Oral dicloxacillin	500 mg every 6 hours	
Oral cephalexin	500 mg every 6 hours	
Oral clindamycin	450 mg every 6 hours	
IV nafcillin	2 grams IV every 4 hours	
IV cefazolin	1 gram IV every 8 hours	
MRSA treatment, oral: clindamycin	450 mg every 6 hours	Other oral MRSA treatment: trimethoprim, sulfamethoxazole
MRSA treatment, IV: vancomycin	1–2 grams IV every 12 hours	Other IV MRSA treatment: linezolid, tigecycline, daptomycin
Therapeutic ultrasound	2 watts/cm² at 1–3 MHz for 5 minutes daily × 2 days (Ritchie, 2013)	Increases circulation. Use as primary treatment for plugged ducts, engorgement, and mild mastitis. For more significant infectious mastitis, use in combination with antibiotics.

Note. Typical antibiotic treatment course is 7–14 days. IV = intravenous. MRSA = methicillin-resistant *Staphylococcus aureus*.

References

Academy of Breastfeeding Medicine. (2008). ABM clinical protocol #4: mastitis. Revision, May 2008. *Breastfeeding Medicine, 3*(3), 177–180.

American Academy of Family Physicians. (2012). *Breastfeeding* (policy statement). Retrieved from http://www.aafp.org/about/policies/all/breastfeeding.html

American Academy of Pediatrics. (2013). *Breastfeeding.* Retrieved from http://www2.aap.org/breastfeeding/faqsbreastfeeding.html

Amir, L. (2014). ABM clinical protocol #4: Mastitis, revised March 2014. *Breastfeeding Medicine, 9*(5), 239–243.

Barrett, M. E., Heller, M. M., Stone, H. F., & Murase, J. E. (2013). Raynaud phenomenon of the nipple in breastfeeding mothers: An underdiagnosed cause of nipple pain. *JAMA Dermatology, 149*(3), 300–306.

Brand, E., Kothari, C., & Stark, M. A. (2011). Factors related to breastfeeding discontinuation between hospital discharge and 2 weeks postpartum. *The Journal of Perinatal Education, 20*(1), 36–44.

Centers for Disease Control and Prevention. (2006). Racial and socioeconomic disparities in breastfeeding—United States, 2004. *MMWR, 55*(12), 335–339.

Centers for Disease Control and Prevention. (2013). *Breastfeeding report cards.* Retrieved from http://www.cdc.gov/breastfeeding/data/reportcard.htm

Chakrabarti, K., & Basu, S. (2011). Management of flat or inverted nipples with simple rubber bands. *Breastfeeding Medicine, 6*(4), 215–219.

Chung, M., Ip, S., Yu, W., Raman, G., Trikalinos, T., DeVine, D., & Lau, J. (2008). Interventions in primary care to promote breastfeeding: A systematic review. In *U.S. Preventive Services Task Force Evidence Syntheses, formerly Systematic Evidence Reviews* (Vol. Oct. Report No.: 09-05126-EF-1.). Rockville, MD: Agency for Healthcare Research and Quality.

Committee on Health Care for Underserved Women, American College of Obstetricians and Gynecologists (2007). ACOG committee opinion No. 361: Breastfeeding: maternal and infant aspects. *Obstetrics and Gynecology, 109*(2 Pt 1), 479–480.

Crepinsek, M. A., Crowe, L., Michener, K., & Smart, N. A. (2010). Interventions for preventing mastitis after childbirth. *The Cochrane Database of Systematic Reviews,* (8), CD007239.

Department of Child and Adolescent Health and Development. (2000). *Mastitis: Causes and management.* Retrieved from http://www.whqlibdoc.who.int/hq/2000/WHO_FCH_CAH_00.13.pdf

Foxman, B., D'Arcy, H., Gillespie, B., Bobo, J. K., & Schwartz, K. (2002). Lactation mastitis: Occurrence and medical management among 946 breastfeeding women in the United States. *American Journal of Epidemiology, 155,* 103–114.

French, L. (2005). POEMs: Fathers can promote breastfeeding. *American Family Physician, 71*(3), 563–564.

Heck, K. E., Braveman, P., Cubbin, C., Chávez, G. F., & Kiely, J. L. (2006). Socioeconomic status and breastfeeding initiation among California mothers. *Public Health Reports, 121*(1), 51–59.

Ip, S., Chung, M., Raman, G., Chew, P., Magula, N., DeVine, D., . . . Lau, J. (2007). Breastfeeding and maternal and infant health outcomes in developed countries. *Evidence Report/Technology Assessment,* (153), 1–186.

Jahanfar, S., Ng, C., & Teng, C. (2013). Antibiotics for mastitis in breastfeeding women. *Cochrane Database of Systematic Reviews,* (2), CD005458.

La Leche League International. (2008). *My doctor said I have inverted or flat nipples. Can I still breastfeed my baby?* Retrieved from http://www.llli.org/faq/flat.html

Lawrence, R. A., & Lawrence, R. M. (1999). *Breastfeeding: A guide for the medical profession* (5th ed.). St. Louis, MO: Mosby

Li, R., Darling, N., Maurice, E., Barker, L., & Grummer-Strawn, L. M. (2005). Breastfeeding rates in the United States by characteristics of the child, mother, or family: The 2002 National Immunization Survey. *Pediatrics, 115*(1), e31–e37.

Livingstone, V. (1997). *Breastfeeding and sore nipples*. Medicine North America.

Mallory, J. (2008). Supplement sampler: *Natural galactogogues*. Retrieved from http://www.fammed.wisc.edu/files/webfmuploads/documents/outreach/im/ss_galactogogues.pdf

Morland-Schultz, K., & Hill, P. D. (2005). Prevention of and therapies for nipple pain: A systematic review. *Journal of Obstetric, Gynecologic & Neonatal Nursing, 34*(4), 428–437. http://dx.doi.org/10.1177/0884217505276056

National Center for Health Statistics & Centers for Disease Control and Prevention. (2011). *Health, United States, 2010: With special feature on death and dying* (Vol. 2013). Hyatssville, MD: Author.

Office of the Surgeon General, Centers for Disease Control and Prevention, & Office on Women's Health. (2011). Barriers to breastfeeding in the United States: *The surgeon general's call to action to support breastfeeding*. Rockville, MD: Office of the Surgeon General.

Office on Women's Health, U.S. Department of Health and Human Services, & Womenshealth.gov. (2011). *Breastfeeding*. Retrieved from http://www.womenshealth.gov/breastfeeding/why-breastfeeding-is-important/

Ritchie, J. (2013). I make milk, what's your superpower?: *The ultimate survival guide to breastfeeding*. Pennsauken, NJ: BookBaby.

Rosen-Carole, C., & Hartman, S. (2015). ABM Clinical Protocol #19: Breastfeeding promotion in the prenatal setting, revision 2015. *Breastfeeding Medicine, 10*(10), 451–457.

Ryan, A., Zhou, W., & Arensberg, M. (2006). The effect of employment status on breastfeeding in the United States. *Womens Health Issues, 16*(5), 243–251.

Weng, S. F., Redsell, S. A., Nathan, D., Swift, J. A., Yang, M., & Glazebrook, C. (2013). Estimating overweight risk in childhood from predictors during infancy. *Pediatrics, 132*(2), e414–e421.

World Health Organization. *Breastfeeding*. Retrieved from http://www.who.int/topics/breastfeeding/en/

World Health Organization. Global Health Observatory Data
  Repository: *Exclusive breastfeeding under 6 months data by WHO
  region.* Retrieved from http://apps.who.int/gho/data/view.main.
  NUT1710?lang=en

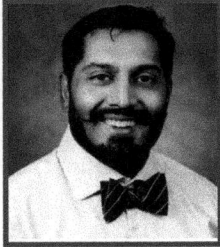

Dr. Khan earned his BA in Philosophy and his BS in Neurobiology, Physiology and Behavior from University of California, Davis. He went on to earn his MD from the University of Washington with a certificate in the Underserved Pathway. Dr. Khan completed his residency training at Harbor-UCLA in family medicine and an obstetrics fellowship at the University of Southern California. He worked in South Central Los Angeles for 2 years and then joined faculty at Ventura in 2014. His clinical interests include high risk obstetrics, breastfeeding support and intervention, inpatient medicine, street and international medicine, and quality improvement.

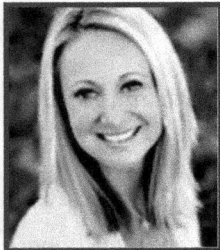

Jennifer received her training through University of California, San Diego and is associated with the Orange County Breastfeeding Coalition. She has two children (both she successfully breastfed) and has helped hundreds of patients through her years as an IBCLC.

USLCA

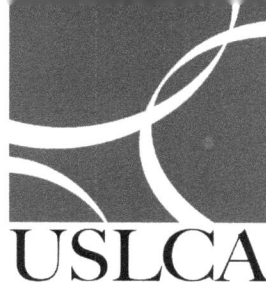

Mammary Dysbiosis

An Unwelcome Visitor During Lactation

Marsha Walker, RN, IBCLC, RLCa

Keywords: bacteriotherapy; probiotics;
mammary dysbiosis; mastitis; subacute mastitis

Mastitis can be an unwelcome and debilitating visitor to breastfeeding mothers. The mammary gland has its own microbiome that can be affected by reduced polymorphonuclear neutrophil recruitment during the first 3 months postpartum, as well as the receipt of antibiotics during the last trimester of pregnancy. This can leave the breast vulnerable to pathologic bacterial over- growth. Mammary dysbiosis is a process whereby the population of potential pathogens increases at the expense of the normal mammary microbiota. Multiresistance to antibiotics plus tricky evasion techniques engaged in by bacterial agents can result in microbes that are elusive to anti-biotic therapy. Therefore, new strategies are needed for the treatment of this threat to continued breastfeeding. Bacteriotherapy, targeting harmless bacteria to displace pathologic organisms, is an emerging therapeutic intervention that uses probiotics instead of antibiotics. Once more high-quality clinical trials of strain-specific probiotics have been conducted, bacteriotherapy may move into mainstream mastitis treatment.

The human body is host to trillions of bacteria that occupy various locations. The totality of microorganisms (such as bacteria, fungi, and viruses) that inhabit a particular environment, their genetic elements, and their environmental interactions is called the microbiome. Frequently seen in breastfeeding discussions are descriptions of the infant gut microbiome, especially how breast milk and infant formula ingestion result in differences in the microbiota that inhabit the gut (Madan et al., 2016). However, both breast milk and the breast tissue itself also have their own microbiome.

Traditionally, human milk was thought to be sterile, and clinicians often went to great lengths to assure that mothers washed their hands and disinfected their nipples before putting the baby to the breast. In 2003, studies began describing the presence of physiological microbiota or normal bacterial residents in human milk (Heikkilä & Saris, 2003; Martín et al., 2003). Early life is when the adult microbiome is established, with the development of the infant gut microbiome occurring along a well-choreographed path directed in large part by the bacteria present in breast milk. It has also been shown that 27.7% of infant gut bacteria are provided by breast milk, and 10.4% of infant gut bacteria are derived from areolar skin (Pannaraj et al., 2017).

Just as breast milk is not sterile, neither is breast tissue. The breast is primarily composed of glandular and fatty tissue. The microbiome of the breast is distinct from the skin and other body sites, with breast tissue housing a diverse community of bacteria. In a study that collected tissue samples from a variety of locations in the breast, it was shown that numerous taxa were present, both health-conferring and pathogenic bacteria (Urbaniak et al., 2014). Bacteria have been isolated in the ducts and lobules in both the lactating and nonlactating breast, but not yet in the fatty tissue (Urbaniak, Burton, & Reid, 2012). Researchers have proposed that the breast microbiome contributes to maintenance of healthy breast tissue by stimulating resident immune cells (Xuan et al., 2014), allowing the breasts' army of defenders to work together to protect the breast.

Where Do These Bacteria Come From?

There are several potential origins and mechanisms thought to be responsible for bacterial presence in the breast.

» Bacteria from the nipple and areola could enter the breast through the nipple pores.

» Bacteria from the infant's mouth could enter the breast during milk backflow. Milk that is not extracted by the infant has been seen on ultrasound to reverse course and flow back into the milk duct (Ramsay et al., 2006).

» Bacteria can enter the breast through a break in the nipple epithelium when a crack or other damage is present.

» Bacterial translocation from the maternal gut to the breast. During pregnancy and lactation, it is believed that bacteria-carrying dendritic cells migrate out of the messenteric lymph nodes in the intestines and into the mammary glands (Urbaniak et al., 2012). This is often referred to as the entero-mammary pathway.

All these routes can contribute to the transport of bacteria to various locations within the breast. The complex ductal system in the breast favors the growth of *S. aureus* and *S. epidermidis*, common residents, but also major contributors to mastitis. Mastitis can be a debilitating intruder on lactation and occurs in up to one-third of breastfeeding women (Foxman, D'Arcy, Gillespie, Bobo, & Schwartz, 2002).

Who Are the Culprits in Acute and Sub-acute Mastitis?

Acute Mastitis

S. aureus is the main etiologic contributor to acute mastitis (Delgado et al., 2011). Under the right conditions, it can proliferate and produce toxins that result in a strong inflammation in the breast tissue. This leads to local intense symptoms of redness, heat, and pain. The toxins are rapidly absorbed into the bloodstream, leading to the systemic flu-like symptoms of fever, muscular pain, and general malaise.

Subacute Mastitis

Coagulase-negative staphylococci (*S. epidermidis*) and viridans streptococci are normal inhabitants in the breast and form thin biofilms that line the ducts, allow normal milk flow, and are swept along during the milk-ejection reflex. Under certain circumstances, overgrowth of these species can occur, leading to subacute or subclinical mastitis. These bacteria do not produce the toxins that are responsible for the debilitating flu-like symptoms of acute mastitis, and the symptoms are generally milder. However, these bacteria can form thick biofilms inside the ducts, inflaming the epithelium, and narrowing the duct so that milk has more difficulty passing through it.

The increasing pressure on the inflamed epithelium is felt as a characteristic needle-like pain, breast cramps, and a burning feeling. These bacterial biofilms may even totally fill some ducts, blocking milk flow, and leading to breast engorgement (Fernández et al., 2014).

If left unchecked, milk production may be reduced, and continued discomfort could lead to premature weaning. These symptoms are frequently attributed to candidiasis and treated with antifungals rather than explored further to discover if the symptoms are actually a manifestation of subacute mastitis. Incorrect antifungal treatment may delay appropriate interventions or exacerbate subacute mastitis. Subacute mastitis is characterized by an elevated sodium/potassium ratio in breast milk and an increased concentration of interlukin-8 (an inflammatory marker; Tuaillon et al., 2017). In a study that collected 110 milk samples during the first month postpartum from healthy mothers with no signs or symptoms of mastitis, subacute mastitis (increased inflammatory factors, an elevated sodium/potassium ratio, and markers of an immune response to bacterial exposure) was seen in 23% of the women (Tuaillon et al., 2017). Subacute mastitis is seen more frequently than acute mastitis and may be a precursor to or the initial stage of inflammation that poses an increased risk of progression to acute or clinical mastitis.

Thus, *S. aureus* is suited to develop acute infections, while *S. epidermidis* is typically the villain in subacute and chronic or recurrent mastitis (Angelopoulou et al.,

2018). When staph and strep are under stress, they form organized and densely populated collectives on epithelia called biofilms. These develop protective coats that resist antibiotics and the host's immune response, allowing rampant bacterial multiplication. Even though these types of bacteria normally reside in the breast in a state of mutual acceptance or tolerance, disturbance of the balanced state between nonpathologic and pathologic bacteria can tip the balance toward mastitis. The ability to cause an infection depends on the strain of the bacteria, how virulent it is, its resistance to antibiotics, its ability to form biofilms, and the presence of other mechanisms that allow it to evade the body's immune response.

Susceptibility to mastitis may also be related to several other contributors, such as the blood group of the mother and the corresponding types of human milk oligosaccharides in her milk. The balanced state of microbes in the breast can be significantly disrupted by intrapartum antibiotics given to the mother, such as during a cesarean delivery or for group B strep prevention. The dysbiosis caused by the antibiotics may result in the loss of lactobacilli and bifidobacterial with the corresponding overgrowth of mastitis-causing agents. Milk that has been depleted of lactobacilli and bifidobacteria, important players in programming the infant gut microbiome, is then delivered to the baby, resulting in alterations of the baby's gut microflora. Women who received antibiotics in the last trimester of pregnancy and peripartum have 25-fold risk of developing mastitis (Bergmann, Rodríguez, Salminen, & Szajewska, 2014).

TABLE 1. Effects of Mastitis on Milk Quantity and Quality	
Selected Factors Thought to be Associated With or Contribute to Mastitis	
Cracked nipples	Oversupply of breast milk
Plugged ducts	Use of nipple shields
Use of breast pumps	Engorgement
Pacifier and bottle use	Milk stasis
Nipple creams	Nipple bleb
Tight bras and clothing	Poor latch
History of mastitis in previous lactations	Fatigue (holidays)
Use of antibiotics and antifungals	Colonized infant

Large amounts of lactose and oligosaccharides are present in breast milk. Both Staphylococcus and Streptococcus are efficient lactose/galactose utilizers. Mammary polymorphonuclear neutrophil recruitment is decreased in first 3 months postpartum so not enough of these leukocytes (immune cells) may be available for control of mastitis-causing bacteria during the early weeks of lactation (Bergmann et al., 2014). This is congruent with peak mastitis occurrence seen during the first 6 weeks postpartum (Foxman et al., 2002). While a number of other factors have been associated with mastitis or thought to be the cause (Cullinane et al., 2015; Table 1), dysbiosis caused by microbial factors (overgrowth of pathogenic bacteria, virulence, biofilm formation, antibiotic resistance), host factors (genetic susceptibility, Lewis antigens, human milk oligosaccharides, autoimmune thyroid disease), and medical factors (antibiotic use, cracked nipples) seems to be the underlying entity responsible for both acute and subacute mastitis (Fernández et al., 2014).

Effects of Mastitis on Milk Quantity and Quality

Inflammatory factors in the mastitic breast can change the metabolic activity of milk-producing cells with the resulting reduction in milk synthesis (Say et al., 2016). Edema of the interstitial tissues is facilitated by the opening of paracellular pathways due to protein leakage from blood and milk. This opening increases the sodium and chloride passage into the milk giving it a salty taste and decreases the potassium and lactose content of the milk. Milk stasis may contribute to the observation of white granules in the milk, which are formed from caseins hardened by salts. Fatty or fibrous-looking material can sometimes be seen in the milk (may look like milk clumps). Fat, carbohydrate, and energy levels have been shown to be significantly lower in the milk from a breast with mastitis (Say et al., 2016). These effects on the quantity and quality of milk may mean that mothers with acute mastitis receive a recommendation to breastfeed more frequently during the course of the mastitis. If the baby will not nurse from the affected breast because of the salty taste of the milk or reduced flow and volume, then that breast will need to be pumped to support ongoing milk production.

Therapeutic Interventions

Antibiotics

Antibiotic therapy (typically dicloxacillin, flucloxacillin, cephalexin, clindamycin) has been the traditional treatment for lactation-related mastitis. However, multidrug resistance to antibiotics and the ability to form biofilms as an evasion technique are hallmark abilities of *S. aureus* and *S. epidermidis*. These two skills explain why mastitis can be a recurrent or chronic infection. In a study looking at antibiotic resistance patterns of human mastitis pathogens, it was found that a remarkable percentage of Staphylococcus isolates (>90%) were resistant to at least one antibiotic (Marín, Arroyo, Espinosa-Martos, Fernández, & Rodríguez, 2017). It has been reported that 25% of mothers who abandon breastfeeding due to mastitis have already received antibiotics (cloxacillin, clindamycin, amoxicillin–clavulanic acid, and/or erythromycin) for 2–4 weeks without resolution (Jiménez et al., 2008).

As an alternative to antibiotic use, and in an effort to avoid therapy failure, disruption of the maternal and infant gut microbiome and dysbiosis in the breast microbiome, probiotic therapy has emerged as a new strategy for the treatment of mastitis. Certain bacteria isolated from human milk have been identified as safe and suitable for therapeutic use in the treatment of mastitis as they have the ability to inhibit bacteria such as *S. aureus* (Heikkilä & Saris, 2003).

Probiotics

Due to the escalating problem of antibiotic resistance, bacteriotherapy, using harmless bacteria to displace pathogenic microorganisms, is being increasingly utilized as a means of combatting bacterial infections. Discussed since the beginning of the 20th century, bacteriotherapy is being utilized for infections in numerous areas of the body, including the breasts. It is important to note that bacteria are commonly referred to by their genus and species names, printed in italics. Strains are a genetic variant or subtype of a microorganism and are designated by strain numbers consisting of several capital letters (the lab where they were constructed) and serial numbering of the strain as a "bookkeeping" method for scientific accuracy and to avoid confusing one mutant with another. In a discussion of probiotics for the treatment of mastitis, only certain strains of a bacterium have been shown to possess specific properties that are effective against the malady.

In 2008, a small pilot trial of 20 women with mastitis, two lactobacilli strains isolated from breast milk were studied as a treatment for Staphylococcal mastitis (Jiménez et al., 2008). Ten mothers received *Lactobacillus salivarius* CECT5713 and *L. gasseri* CECT5714 (10 log10 CFU of each) for a 4-week period, while the other 10 mothers received a placebo. By day 14, clinical signs of mastitis were no longer observed in the probiotic group, while mastitis persisted in the control group. In a larger study of 352 women with mastitis, one group received *Lactobacillus fermentum* CECT5716, one group received *L. salivarius* CECT5713, and a third group received antibiotic therapy (Arroyo et al., 2010). At the end of the 21-day trial, mothers in both probiotic groups had either recovered completely or experienced only slight breast discomfort compared to the antibiotic group where intense pain or breast discomfort persisted for the entire course of antibiotics. The rate of recurrence of mastitis was significantly higher in the antibiotic group. Seeking to discover if varying doses of probiotics would differentially lower the load of *Staphylococcus* in breast milk of women with subacute mastitis and reduce pain levels, a study evaluated the effect of three different escalating doses of *L. fermentum* CECT5716 (Maldonado-Lobónet al., 2015). All three doses lowered Staphylococcus levels in breast milk and significantly reduced pain by 30%. A dose–response effect was not seen.

In an effort to prevent mastitis by the prophylactic use of probiotics, two studies explored using probiotics either during pregnancy or for 16 weeks postpartum. In a study of 108 pregnant women who had experienced mastitis after at least one previous pregnancy, one group was given daily oral capsules of *L. salivarius* PS2 from 30 weeks of pregnancy until birth, and the control group received a placebo from 30 weeks of pregnancy until birth (Fernández et al., 2016). Of the 108 women, 41% developed mastitis, 25% in the probiotic group and 57% in the control group, a 56% decrease in mastitis incidence. When mastitis occurred, the milk bacterial counts in the probiotic group were significantly lower than those in the placebo group. In a study of 291 women from birth until 16 weeks, one group received the probiotic *L. fermentum* CECT5716, and one group received a placebo (Hurtado et al., 2017). In the probiotic group, 16 women developed mastitis, while 30 women in the control group did. This represents a 51% reduction in the incidence rate of clinical mastitis in the group taking probiotics. Specific strains of probiotics seem to be demonstrating themselves as an efficient strategy to prevent mastitis in breastfeeding mothers.

Bacteriocins

Bacteriocins are antimicrobial peptides (short amino acid chains) produced by one bacterium that are active against other bacteria, either in the same species (narrow spectrum) or across genera (broad spectrum). They exhibit potent activity against other bacteria, including antibiotic-resistant strains. Many bacteriocins are produced by lactic acid bacteria. Lantibiotics are a group of bacteriocins, one of which is nisin.

Nisin is produced by certain strains of *Lactococcus lactis*, a common species found in breast milk of healthy women. One use of nisin is as an antimicrobial in the food industry to prevent spoilage in food from pathogens and food spoilage microorganisms. It has also been used in the dairy industry to treat bovine mastitis. Nisin was investigated for use in treating infectious mastitis in breastfeeding mothers in a small 2-week study of women who had already received antibiotics for 2 to 4 weeks, but which failed to remedy the infection (Fernández, Delgado, Herrero, Maldonado, & Rodríguez, 2008). One group of mothers applied a topical solution of 0.1 mL nisin to their nipples and areolae after each feeding, while the control group applied a placebo solution. *Staphylococcal* counts in the nisin group were significantly lower after 2 weeks. Clinical symptoms were notably improved in the nisin group by day 7, with the complete disappearance of local inflammation and flu-like symptoms by day 14. In contrast, clinical signs remained persistent in the control group for the entire study period.

Topical Treatment for Inflammation

Markers for mastitis, such as breast pain, breast tension, and erythema (redness) are not uncommon in breast-feeding women and may represent the initial entrance into the mastitis continuum. Seeking alternative treatments to antibiotics, one study was conducted to determine the efficacy of topical curcumin (turmeric) in reducing breast inflammation, as curcumin is known to have anti-inflammatory properties (Afshariani, Farhadi, Ghaffarpasand, & Roozbeh, 2014). A randomized, double-blind clinical trial was conducted with 70 breastfeeding mothers suffering from breast pain, breast tension, and erythema. The experimental group applied one pump of Curcumin Cream-200 mg (Neurobiologix, TX, USA) to the affected breast every 8 hours for 3 days. At the end of 72 hours of therapy, the curcumin group had significantly decreased markers of lactational mastitis such as pain, breast tension, and erythema compared to the control group.

TABLE 2. Overview of Some Mastitis Treatment Options
Antibiotics (Amir & Academy of Breastfeeding Medicine Protocol Committee, 2014)
If conservative management does not improve symptoms within 24 hours or mother is acutely ill.
• Dicloxacillin (penicillinase-resistant penicillin)
• Flucloxacillin (penicillinase-resistant penicillin)
• Cephalexin (mother allergic to penicillin)
• Clindamycin (mother with severe penicillin allergy)
• Vancomycin or trimethoprim/sulfamethoxazole (if mastitis is not improving after 48 hours of treatment and methicillin-resistant *S. aureus* (MRSA) have been confirmed.
Probiotics
As an alternative or complement to antibiotic therapy; as a preventive measure; as first-line therapy for subacute mastitis; as conservative management if mastitis symptoms are mild and have been present for less than 24 hours.
• *L. salivarius* PS2—as a preventive measure, 9 $\log_{10}$ CFU daily from 30 weeks of pregnancy until delivery
• *L. fermentum* CECT5716—as a preventive measure, 3 $\log_{10}$ CFU daily from birth to 16 weeks postpartum
• *L. fermentum* CECT5716—as a first-line treatment of confirmed acute mastitis, 9 $\log_{10}$ CFU daily for 21 days
• *L. salivarius* CECT5713—as a first-line treatment of confirmed acute mastitis, 9 $\log_{10}$ CFU daily for 21 days
Bacteriocins
As an alternative or complement to antibiotics
• *L. lactis* ESI515 as the source for nisin—topical nisin solution (0.1 mL) applied to the nipple and areola after each breastfeeding for 14 days for treatment of acute mastitis
Topical Curcumin
For relief of inflammation and breast pain in subacute mastitis
• Curcumin—200 mg cream applied to the breast every 8 hours for 3 days

Where Do We Go From Here?

Bacteriotherapy represents a promising addition to our toolbox of mastitis treatment options (Table 2).

While this is an exciting possibility, bacteriotherapy is still an emerging treatment option. The best treatment option for mastitis is prevention by prompt and sound lactation management from skilled clinicians. Mastitis can be thought of as a continuum from plugged ducts and engorgement to cracked nipples, subacute mastitis, and acute mastitis. Interruption of the continuum is a desirable goal to avoid the occurrence of mastitis altogether. Despite the need for more clinical trials (Amir, Griffin, Cullinane, & Garland, 2016), several of the studied probiotics have reached the market and are available for mothers to use. It is important to note that only the specific probiotic strains that have been shown to be effective are possibilities for mastitis treatment. A mother's healthcare team would need to evaluate if and how such therapy would be appropriate as well as if bacteriotherapy were administered exclusively or in conjunction with antibiotics. Several of the studied probiotics are commercially available:

» Lactanza hereditum (Angelini, Barcelona, Spain)

» Qiara (Puremedic, Kew, Victoria, Australia)

» Target b2 (Klaire Labs, Reno, Nevada, USA)

Random probiotic supplements on store shelves that have not been evaluated as therapeutic agents for mastitis are not recommended for such use. Once more high-quality clinical trials of strain-specific probiotics have been conducted, bacteriotherapy may move into mainstream mastitis treatment, a most welcome event.

References

Afshariani, R., Farhadi, P., Ghaffarpasand, F., & Roozbeh, J. (2014). Effectiveness of topical curcumin for treatment of mastitis in breastfeeding women: A randomized, double-blind, placebo-controlled clinical trial. *Oman Medical Journal, 29*(5), 330–334. http://dx.doi.org/10.5001/omj.2014.89

Amir, L. H., & Academy of Breastfeeding Medicine Protocol Committee (2014). ABM clinical protocol #4: Mastitis, revised March 2014. *Breastfeeding Medicine, 9*(5), 239–243. http://dx.doi.org/10.1089/bfm.2014.9984

Amir, L. H., Griffin, L., Cullinane, M., & Garland, S. M. (2016). Probiotics and mastitis: Evidence-based marketing? *International Breastfeeding Journal, 11*, 19. http://dx.doi.org/10.1186/s13006-016-0078-5

Angelopoulou, A., Field, D., Ryan, C. A., Stanton, C., Hill, C., & Ross, R. P. (2018). The microbiology and treatment of human mastitis. *Medical Microbiology and Immunology, 207*(2), 83–94. http://dx.doi.org/10.1007/s00430-017-0532-z

Arroyo, R., Martín, V., Maldonado, A., Jiménez, E., Fernández, L., & Rodríguez, J. M. (2010). Treatment of infectious mastitis during lactation: Antibiotics versus oral administration of lactobacilli isolated from breast milk. *Clinical Infectious Diseases, 50*(12), 1551–1558. http://dx.doi.org/10.1086/652763

Bergmann, H., Rodríguez, J. M., Salminen, S., & Szajewska, H. (2014). Probiotics in human milk and probiotic supplementation in infant nutrition: A workshop report. *British Journal of Nutrition, 112*(7), 1119–1128. http://dx.doi.org/10.1017/S0007114514001949

Cullinane, M., Amir, L. H., Donath, S. M., Garland, S. M., Tabrizi, S. N., Payne, M. S., & Bennett, C. M. (2015). Determinants of mastitis in women in the CASTLE study: A cohort study. *BMC Family Practice, 16*, 181. http://dx.doi.org/10.1186/s12875-015-0396-5

Delgado, S., García, P., Fernández, L., Jiménez, E., Rodríguez-Baños, M., del Campo, R., & Rodríguez, J. M. (2011). Characterization of Staphylococcus aureus strains involved in human and bovine mastitis. *FEMS Immunology & Medical Microbiology, 62*(2), 225–235. http://dx.doi.org/10.1111/j.1574695X.2011.00806.x

Fernández, L., Arroyo, R., Espinosa, I., Marín, M., Jiménez, E., & Rodríguez, J. M. (2014). Probiotics for human lactational mastitis. *Beneficial Microbes, 5*(2), 169–183. http://dx.doi.org/10.3920/BM2013.0036

Fernández, L., Cárdenas, N., Arroyo, R., Manzano, S., Jiménez, E., Martín, V., & Rodríguez, J. M. (2016). Prevention of infectious mastitis by oral administration of Lactobacillus salivarius PS2 during late pregnancy. *Clinical Infectious Diseases, 62*(5), 568–573. http://dx.doi.org/10.1093/cid/civ974

Fernández, L., Delgado, S., Herrero, H., Maldonado, A., & Rodríguez, J. M. (2008). The bacteriocin nisin, an effective agent for the treatment of staphylococcal mastitis during lactation. *Journal of Human Lactation, 24*(3), 311–316. http://dx.doi.org/10.1177/0890334408317435

Foxman, B., D'Arcy, H., Gillespie, B., Bobo, J. K., & Schwartz, K. (2002). Lactation mastitis: Occurrence and medical management among 946 breastfeeding women in the United States. *American Journal of Epidemiology, 155*(2), 103–114. http://dx.doi.org/10.1093/aje/155.2.103

Heikkilä, M. P., & Saris, P. E. (2003). Inhibition of Staphylococcus aureus by the commensal bacteria of human milk. *Journal of Applied Microbiology, 95*(3), 471–478. http://dx.doi.org/10.1046/j.1365-2672.2003.02002.x

Hurtado, J. A., Maldonado-Lobón, J. A., Díaz-Ropero, M. P., Flores-Rojas, K., Uberos, J., Leante, J. L., . . . the PROLAC Group. (2017). Oral administration to nursing women of Lactobacillus fermentum CECT5716 prevents lactational mastitis development: A randomized controlled trial. *Breastfeeding Medicine, 12*(4), 202–209. http://dx.doi.org/10.1089/bfm.2016.0173

Jiménez, E., Fernández, L., Maldonado, A., Martín, R., Olivares, M., Xaus, J., & Rodríguez, J. M. (2008). Oral administration of Lactobacillus strains isolated from breast milk as an alternative for the treatment of infectious mastitis during lactation. *Applied and Environmental Microbiology, 74*(15), 4650–4655. http://dx.doi.org/10.1128/AEM.02599-07

Madan, J. C., Hoen, A. G., Lundgren, S. N., Farzan, S. F., Cottingham, K. L., Morrison, H. G., . . . Karagas, M. R. (2016). Association of cesarean delivery and formula supplementation with the intestinal microbiome of 6-week-old infants. *JAMA Pediatrics, 170*(3), 212–219. http://dx.doi.org/10.1001/jamapediatrics.2015.3732

Maldonado-Lobón, J. A., Díaz-López, M. A., Carputo, R., Duarte, P., Díaz-Ropero, M. P., Valero, A. D., . . . Olivares Martín, M. (2015). Lactobacillus fermentum CECT 5716 Reduces Staphylococcus load in the breastmilk of lactating mothers suffering breast pain: A randomized controlled trial. *Breastfeeding Medicine, 10*(9), 425–432. http://dx.doi.org/10.1089/bfm.2015.0070

Martín, R., Langa, S., Reviriego, C., Jimínez, E., Marín, M. L., Xaus, J., . . . Rodríguez, J. M. (2003). Human milk is a source of lactic acid bacteria for the infant gut. *The Journal of Pediatrics, 143*(6), 754–758. http://dx.doi.org/10.1016/j.jpeds.2003.09.028

Marín, M., Arroyo, R., Espinosa-Martos, I., Fernández, L., & Rodríguez, J. M. (2017). Identification of emerging human mastitis pathogens by MALDI-TOF and assessment of their antibiotic resistance patterns. *Frontiers in Microbiology, 8*, 1258. http://dx.doi.org/10.3389/fmicb.2017.01258

Pannaraj, P. S., Li, F., Cerini, C., Bender, J. M., Yang, S., Rollie, A., . . . Aldrovandi, G. M. (2017). Association between breast milk bacterial communities and establishment and development of the infant gut microbiome. *JAMA Pediatrics, 171*(7), 647–654. http://dx.doi.org/10.1001/jamapediatrics.2017.0378

Ramsay, D. T., Mitoulas, L. R., Kent, J. C., Cregan, M. D., Doherty, D. A., Larsson, M., & Hartmann, P. E. (2006). Milk flow rates can be used to identify and investigate milk ejection in women expressing breast milk using an electric breast pump. *Breastfeeding Medicine, 1*(1), 14–23. http://dx.doi.org/10.1089/bfm.2006.1.14

Say, B., Dizdar, E. A., Degirmencioglu, H., Uras, N., Sari, F. N., Oguz, S., & Canpolat, F. E. (2016). The effect of lactational mastitis on the macronutrient content of breast milk. *Early Human Development, 98*, 7–9. http://dx.doi.org/10.1016/j.earlhumdev.2016.03.009

Tuaillon, E., Viljoen, J., Dujols, P., Cambonie, G., Rubbo, P. A., Nagot, N., . . . Van de Perre, P. (2017). Subclinical mastitis occurs frequently in association with dramatic changes in inflammatory/anti-inflammatory breast milk components. *Pediatric Research, 81*(4), 556–564. http://dx.doi.org/10.1038/pr.2016.220

Urbaniak, C., Burton, J. P., & Reid, G. (2012). Breast, milk and microbes: A complex relationship that does not end with lactation. *Women's Health, 8*(4), 385–398. http://dx.doi.org/10.2217/WHE.12.23

Urbaniak, C., Cummins, J., Brackstone, M., Macklaim, J. M., Gloor, G. B., Baban, C. K., . . . Reid, G. (2014). Microbiota of human breast tissue. *Applied and Environmental Microbiology, 80*(10), 3007–3014. http://dx.doi.org/10.1128/AEM.00242-14

Xuan, C., Shamonki, J. M., Chung, A., Dinome, M. L., Chung, M., Sieling, P. A., & Lee, D. J. (2014). Microbial dysbiosis is associated with human breast cancer. *PLoS ONE, 9*(1), e83744. http://dx.doi.org/10.1371/journal.pone.0083744

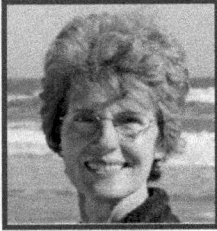

Marsha Walker, RN, IBCLC, RLC, is a registered nurse and IBCLC. She is the executive director of the National Alliance for Breastfeeding Advocacy (NABA) and a previous member of the board of directors of the U.S. Lactation Consultant Association (USLCA), the Massachusetts Breastfeeding Coalition, and Baby Friendly U.S.A. She is USLCA's representative to the USDA's Breastfeeding Promotion Consortium and NABA's representative to the U.S. Breastfeeding Committee. She is an Associate Editor for Clinical Lactation.

Special Section on World Health Assembly Resolution

As reported by *The New York Times* (https://www.nytimes.com/2018/07/08/health/world-health-breastfeeding-ecuador-trump.html), this spring, the U.S. Delegation to the World Health Assembly undermined a global resolution aimed at supporting breastfeeding (http://apps.who.int/gb/ebwha/pdf_files/WHA71/A71_ACONF4Rev1-en.pdf), threatening trade sanctions against Ecuador before yielding to a proposal put forth by Russia Breastfeeding organizations and advocates across the country have raised concerns about the role of industry in international policy and the aggressive tactics of the U.S. delegation. See the Weekly Wire for a list of member and partner statements: http://www.usbreastfeeding.org/p/bl/et/blogid=1&blogaid=2080

Source: USBC

USLCA

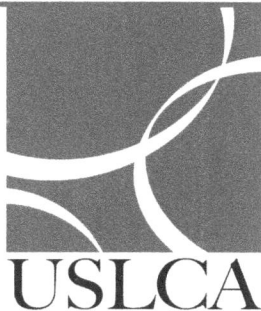

USLCA is a non-profit membership association focused on advancing the International Board Certified Lactation Consultant (IBCLC) in the United States through leadership, advocacy, professional development, and research.

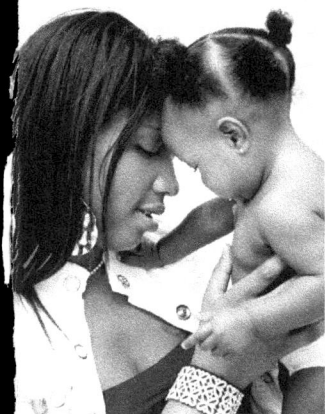

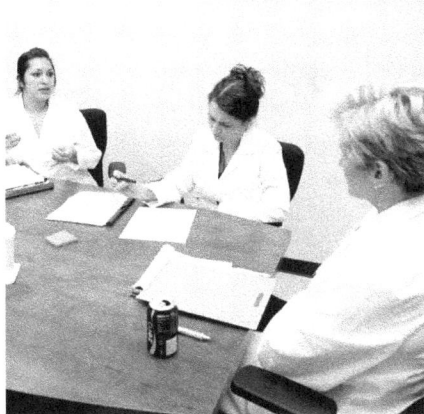

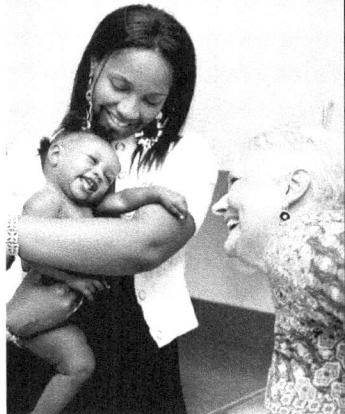

Join USLCA today
202-738-1125 | Washington, D.C. | www.USLCA.org

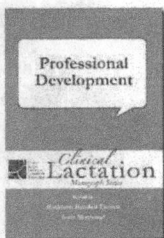

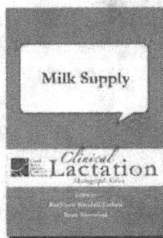

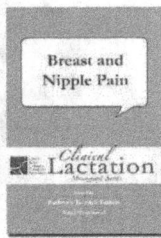

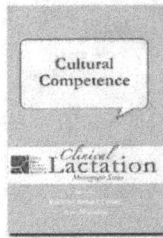

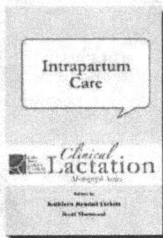

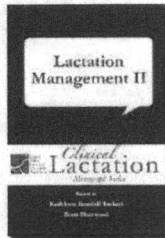

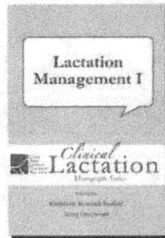

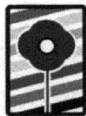

Breastfeeding and Women's Health Titles from Praeclarus Press

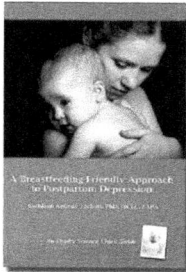

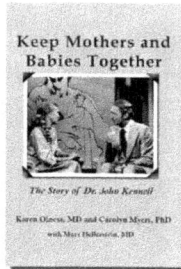

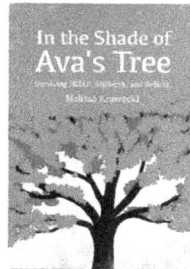

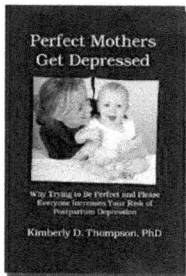

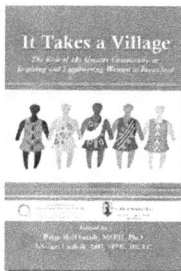

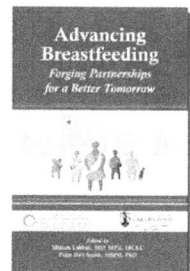

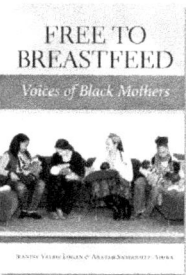

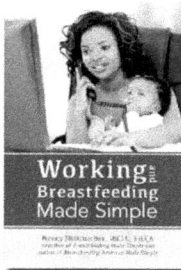

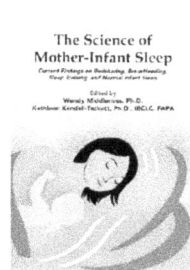

A Breastfeeding-Friendly Approach to Postpartum Depression

Keep Mothers and Babies Together
The Story of Dr. John Kennell
Karen Olness, MD and Carolyn Myers, PhD
with Marc DeBenetta, MD

In the Shade of Ava's Tree
Meltem Krawecki

Perfect Mothers Get Depressed
Why Trying to Be Perfect and Please Everyone Increases Your Risk of Postpartum Depression
Kimberly D. Thompson, PhD

It Takes a Village

Advancing Breastfeeding
Forging Partnerships for a Better Tomorrow

FREE TO BREASTFEED
Voices of Black Mothers

Working and Breastfeeding Made Simple

The Science of Mother-Infant Sleep
Edited by
Wendy Middlemiss, Ph.D.
Kathleen Kendall-Tackett, Ph.D., IBCLC, FAPA

Praeclarus Press
Excellence in Women's Health

www.PraeclarusPress.com

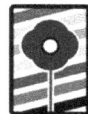

www.ingramcontent.com/pod-product-compliance
Lightning Source LLC
Chambersburg PA
CBHW072013290326
41934CB00007BA/1071